# DISPOSITIONALISM
## *in*
# MUSCULOSKELETAL
## *Care*

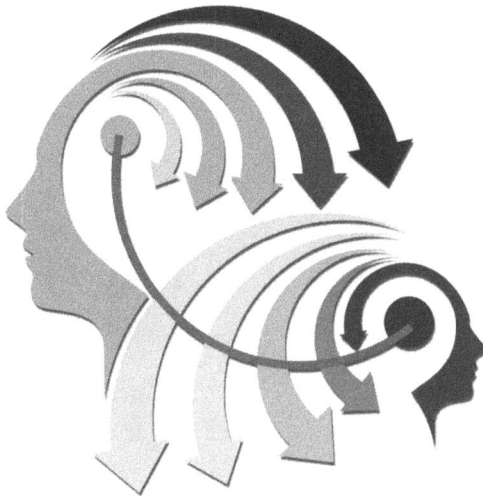

## MICHAEL VIANIN MSc DC

# DISPOSITIONALISM
*in*
# MUSCULOSKELETAL
*Care*

Understanding and Integrating Unique Characteristics
of the Clinical Encounter to Optimize Patient Care

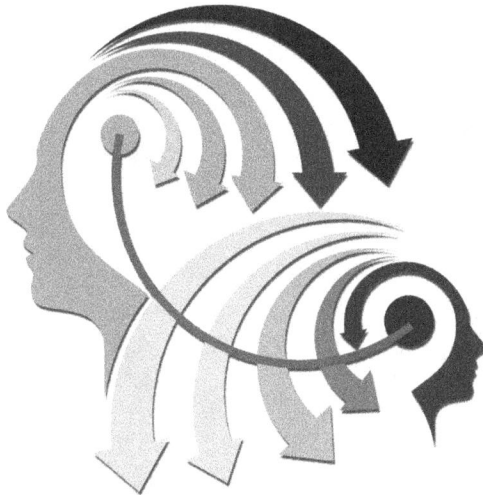

## MICHAEL VIANIN MSc DC

First edition 2021

ISBN (Paperback): 978-0-6452404-3-6
ISBN (eBook): 978-0-6452404-5-0
ISBN (Hardcover): 978-0-6452404-4-3


CONTACT THE PUBLISHER:

Evolve Global Publishing
www.evolveglobalpublishing.com
Interior V5


CONTACT THE AUTHOR:

Michael Vianin
www.mskcarethebook.com
Photo credits: ©Keren Bisaz / Mirages Photography

# Table of Contents

Michael Vianin MSc DC

*To Nathalie. My wife. My best friend.*

*Thank you for showing me the path to authenticity. I love you.*

Michael Vianin MSc DC

# Acknowledgment

A handful of people have influenced my life over the years. It seems someone was always present at the right time to guide me towards the right path when I was facing a crossroads. I am grateful to all these people because they helped shape the person I am. They also all had an impact on my motivation to write this book.

My parents and my big brother, my only sibling, were obviously the ones who had an early impact. My parents taught me things do not fall in someone's lap by chance — you have to work hard to get the things you need or want. They provided my brother and me with loving support and worked really hard to allow us to pursue our studies. They gave us the opportunity to improve ourselves. My brother taught me that even though the path might be full of turns and twists, perseverance always pays off. I am really proud of what he achieved. Thank you.

Next in line are my teachers. Over my long academic career, I have crossed paths with lots of educators but only a few teachers who had a true impact on my life. They believed in me and encouraged me to give it a try and not worry about the non-believers. They challenged me and opened my mind to new knowledge. They gave me advice and carried me through difficult times. They were hard but fair and motivated me to be the best I can be. Thank you.

I should not forget the non-believers who told me things would be too much for me to handle. They made me angry; they made me cry. They also gave me the determination to never give up — to prove them wrong. That willpower carried me through some tough times. Thank you.

My wife, Nathalie. My wife is the most direct and honest person I know. She can be brutally honest — and brutal she has been with me. She taught me that, even as difficult as it seems, total honesty is the best way forward. You might lose some feathers along the way, but you will feel good about yourself and the world around you. She is also the person with the most fortitude I know. She fights and carries on through whatever life throws at her and never complains. She is amazing. I am in total admiration of her resilience. Thank you.

My three kids — Charline, Elise, and Adrien — are rays of sunshine in my life. They are a bunch of energy that invigorates me. They have taught me that every moment counts and we should make the most of the time we have together. They also try to teach me to work less — maybe one day I will learn — and have been very patient during the whole book writing and editing process, even though they missed their dad. Thank you.

My patients. They are the motivating force in my professional life. Every patient teaches me something and pushes me to become a better practitioner. Every clinical encounter helps me understand a little more and motivates me to learn more and to find better ways to help them. Thank you.

All the students I have encountered challenged me to know my stuff inside out and to find answers when I did not know something. Every single one of them also opened my eyes to something new. One truly learns by teaching. Thank you.

This book would certainly not have seen the light of day if not for the guidance and the work of everyone at Evolve Global Publishing. Special thanks to John, Kellie, Leanne, and Maki for their guidance and work, and for putting up with me and my never-ending requests. Thank you.

Last but not least, my book launch team. They provided me with constructive criticism and encouraging words during the book writing process. More than that, they share their friendship with me and each one of them, in their own way, helps me keep things in perspective. Thank you.

# About the Author

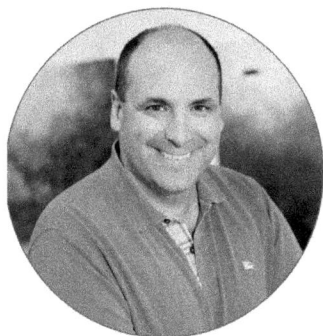

*Michael Vianin (MSc, DC)* is a chiropractor with a Master's degree in Rehabilitation Sciences who has almost twenty years of experience working with people who suffer from musculoskeletal (MSK) pain. He specializes in the management of complex cases, including post-operative care. Michael also has extensive teaching experience in the rehabilitation of MSK disorders and in mentoring interns and residents.

Starting his career as a member of a multidisciplinary spinal pain team in Fribourg in Switzerland, Michael was also a Team Chiropractor with HC Fribourg-Gottéron, a professional, Swiss ice hockey team, and engaged to lecture in Active Rehabilitation at Zurich University's Faculty of Medicine. Michael currently balances his roles as expert examiner and reviewer of Federal Chiropractic Examinations, Team Chiropractor and Head of the Concussion Unit (HC Fribourg-Gottéron), Staff Physician with Clinique Générale, Supervising Clinician with CHUV (University Hospital in Lausanne), and Chiropractic Physician at his own private practice in Fribourg.

Michael has a keen interest in the unique qualities of each of his patients. His drive to continue learning about the clinical usefulness of the impact of patient dispositions on symptoms presentation and treatment outcomes has brought him to share his knowledge and experience with readers through Dispositionalism in Musculoskeletal Care.

Combining his passion for his career with his love for his family and an active, outdoor lifestyle, Michael believes the important lessons in life can come in many different ways. It is only when we have the courage to embrace each moment, keep an open mind to change, and maintain our enthusiasm to learn, that we will reap the benefits of constructive change.

# What Others Say About Michael

*I have worked with Dr. M Vianin for more than twenty years. Over this time, I have appreciated, from a surgical perspective, his high level of competence in the broad field of spinal disease. We collaborate on numerous difficult cases. Michael knows very well all the different therapeutic modalities for spinal diseases, including operative indication, and also follows up with the patients, before and after surgery, offering comfort, security and advice, and leading them through the sometimes difficult re-adaptation. Those patients are extremely grateful for the benefits of their treatment. Dr. Vianin has never ceased to improve his knowledge, reading a lot, with a critical and scientific mind, and always sharing the most recent advances in chiropractic science. It is a privilege to work with Dr. Vianin. I am honoured to be his friend and colleague, and immensely impressed by his dedication to his profession.*

**— Dr. Philippe Otten, Neurosurgeon**

*Michael Vianin is a very empathetic person and an excellent physician. It is both a stroke of luck and an honor for me to be able to work with him. All the athletes I have cared for have been completely satisfied so far. With all of them, there were important points that led to a quick recovery. However, the area of prevention seems much more important to me. So far, we have been able to apply injury-preventive or performance-enhancing measures for all athletes, through good teamwork between the athlete, the physician, and the coach. At this trusting level of cooperation, it is very easy for us to advise and support our clients to their full satisfaction.*

**— Bruno Knutti, professional trainer and sports teacher, consultant and coach**

*I was fortunate to have Dr. Vianin as my supervisor whilst completing my sixth year of Chiropractic Medicine at the CHUV (Centre Hospitalier Universitaire Vaudois, Switzerland) between 2019 and 2020. He was always supportive and eager to help us grow as clinicians. With his clinical experience and depth of knowledge, he constantly made us think critically about our clinical decisions, whilst making it a safe learning environment. I am grateful to have had Dr. Vianin as my supervisor and, thanks to him, I was able to hone my clinical skills and ultimately become a better clinician.*

**— Nils Osseiran, Chiropractic Assistant**

*As Project Manager of the Swiss Federal chiropractic license examination, I have worked with Michael Vianin for the last thirteen years. In that time, I observed him working as an expert in two different teams – one being the group developing the written exam questions and the other being the team developing the practical, objective, structured clinical examination. Team spirit, a sense of responsibility and dedication are some of his strengths. I particularly remember his fairness when stepping into the role as an examiner on the clinical examination.*

*There are a couple of things I know I will miss about him when we no longer work together — his wittiness and agreeableness.*

**— Dr Beatrice Zaugg, Chiropractor**

*I've worked with Michael in the fitness, rehabilitation, and personal trainer education space across three continents since 2006. In that time, I've seen Michael change the lives of quite literally thousands of people. When it comes to getting patients out of pain and correcting biomechanical dysfunction, Michael is by far the best health professional I've ever seen.*

*One thing that I miss is working with Michael on a day-to-day basis and the multidisciplinary approach we applied to our patients and clients. I recommend this book to any health professional who enjoys learning from the best and wants to add value to their own business.*

**— Jason Thomas, CEO and Co-Founder, goXpro International Operations Pty Ltd.**

*I had the chance to study under the supervision of Dr. Michael Vianin at the CHUV (Centre Hospitalier Universitaire Vaudois). He was able to transmit his knowledge with ease and clarity, whilst always taking the time to ensure my progress as a clinician. Thanks to his expertise and his teaching, I became a better clinician.*

— **Laure Béranger, Chiropractic Assistant**

*I've been a regular patient of Dr. Vianin for over 10 years. I had so much tension in my body that it was too difficult for my fitness coach to find suitable exercises for me, so he sent me to Dr. Vianin. I needed a precise report explaining my weaknesses so my fitness coach could adapt my program. This has been very helpful, and I haven't needed any physiotherapist appointments since then. I also have osteopathic appointments from time to time and Dr. Vianin never discouraged me from trying to find solutions elsewhere. He is open-minded enough to collaborate with other types of medicine and isn't like some practitioners who think they are the only ones who can solve their patients' problems. Even if I'm not cured, my general health has clearly improved and I can live without any medicine, which is already amazing.*

*Part of the success of the treatment is due to the doctor's personality and charisma as well. I must admit that his therapeutic methods are sometimes intense, and without the friendly relationship we have built over the years, I would be apprehensive of my appointments.*

*His office is pleasant, and his two secretaries are welcoming and smiling. Everything in the waiting room is made so that I do not think about the pain. Dr. Vianin always welcomes his patients by looking them in the eye, and with a good firm handshake. These are little details, but as a patient, you feel that the doctor is fully present for you from the beginning to the end of the appointment, which is not always the case elsewhere.*

*I am aware that a great part of my physical tension is psychological and that I should change some aspects of my life to get better. Dr. Vianin and I often discuss these factors, but he has never judged me or put pressure on me to change quicker than I could. He really listens to me, and I have always felt understood. Obviously, this does not really change the application of his treatments, but it makes me feel good enough to forget about the pain and to leave the medical practice with a positive state of mind.*

*I met several other chiropractors before Dr. Vianin, but none helped me as much and I feel really lucky to have met him.*

— **Cendrine Maillard, patient**

*In my 15 years as a top athlete, my body always had to perform at a high level. Without the competent and professional support of Dr. Michael Vianin, and especially his gift for precisely identifying the cause of my respective pains - and eliminating them in a targeted manner and within the shortest possible time - I would not have been able to pursue my passion, ice hockey, with the same quality and in such good physical condition.*

**— Marc Abplanalp, professional hockey player**

*In my experience as a student, certain mentors are remembered for the rest of your life. Dr. Vianin was, and still is, a role model for countless reasons. His insatiable thirst for knowledge, his human approach to healthcare, and his pedagogy during educational exchanges are unparalleled, and these are only a few qualities that make him a true inspiration. He is always available to guide and generously continues to pass on his expertise. I can only look forward to reading his work and salute the person and the brain behind the synthesis of a bottomless well of knowledge. Thank you for all you have been.*

**— Adrien Aymon Rose, Chiropractic Assistant**

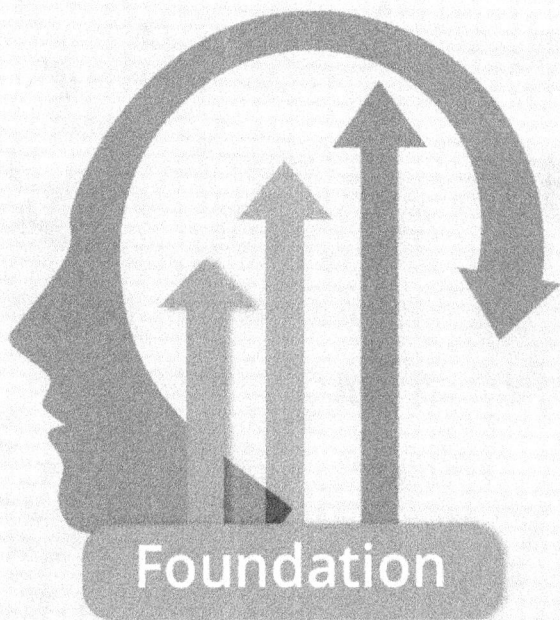

Foundation

# Introduction

Michael Vianin MSc DC

# Change in Paradigm

The global burden that has been associated with chronic and non-communicable diseases is enormous, particularly the conditions associated with morbidity, of which musculoskeletal (MSK) conditions have been ranked among the highest. Common MSK pain conditions, such as neck, back, and joint pain, are the leading cause of disability worldwide.(1)

Despite the large and growing burden and cost to society from MSK conditions, management has relied on an outdated, structural-mechanical, pathology-based model of care, instead of embracing a contemporary, patient-centered, disposition-based model of care. This book aims to focus on newer research and concepts that can assist practitioners in exploring and overcoming the barriers in implementing a change in paradigm.

The *2018 Lancet* Low Back Pain Series acknowledged the gap in the implementation of recommendations from up-to-date, clinical guidelines and proposed solutions for large-scale implementation.(2) An update of the series, published in 2020, concludes that despite the high accessibility and coverage of the 2018 series, improvements in the management of low back pain (LBP) were scarce and that LBP:

- remains the leading global cause of disability
- is associated with heavy direct and indirect costs
- is often incorrectly treated with many patients still receiving the wrong care.(3)

Clinical guidelines for the management of MSK disorders call for an integrative approach to patient care, where the patient is seen as a whole person and not as someone who has a specific disorder. The difficulty in applying these guidelines lies in the conceptualization of disease and illness that has dominated the culture of medicine since the nineteenth century — the biomedical model of illness. The biomedical model sees illness as being reducible to a physical, biological disease.(4),(5) Disease, in turn, is seen as one or more malfunctions at lower structural and functional levels of organisms (e.g. genes, cells, tissues, hormones), that can be measured by deviations of measurable, biological (somatic) variables.(4),(6) The biomedical model relies on a bottom-up causality, where the origin of an illness goes from causes at a lower level of organization to impact a higher level of organization (e.g. a headache caused by hormonal fluctuations).(4)

The biomedical model approach to MSK care has led to massive development and utilization of sophisticated testing technologies to find injured and defective structures to explain patients' complaints. The emergence and utilization of modern diagnostic technologies have led to over-detection, overdiagnosis, and overtreatment of structural anomalies in MSK disorders with overdiagnosis being one of the most harmful and costly problems in modern healthcare.(7) Examples of over-detection and overdiagnosis in MSK care that lead to overtreatment abound:

- Asymptomatic elite-level volleyball players show extensive shoulder pathology on MRI, including rotator cuff tendinosis, partial rotator cuff tears, labral tears, and labral fraying.(8) Furthermore, subacromial decompression surgery shows no additional benefit when compared with placebo surgery or exercise therapy.(9),(10)

- Hip morphology does not correlate with hip symptoms.(11),(12) Labral tears in the hip are found in most (87%) asymptomatic rugby players and ballet dancers, and acetabular cartilage loss is found in more than 50% of the same athletes.(13)

- Knee MRIs of asymptomatic, uninjured knees show features of osteoarthritis in nearly 50% of people over forty.(14) Knee cartilage thickness loss is associated with only a small amount of worsening knee pain.(15) The majority of comparative trials for knee arthroscopic meniscectomy and knee arthroscopic debridement for osteoarthritis did not favor surgery.(10) A considerable number of patients with advanced radiographic knee osteoarthritis do not report pain.(16)

- MRI-confirmed progressive degeneration in lumbar discs over thirty years does not predict pain, disability, or clinical symptoms.(17) Disc degeneration and facet joint degeneration are not associated with long-term disability in patients with chronic LBP.(18) An MRI-confirmed progression of degenerative changes in the cervical spine over twenty years is not associated with clinical symptoms.(19)

MSK care has been plagued by the reductionist biomedical model of illness. The biomedical model of illness has served us well in diseases, such as infections, and has led to great advances in medicine, including the discovery of antibiotics, but it is ill-adapted to serve complex health problems, such as MSK disorders. In such disorders, a patient must be considered as a whole person whose experience is influenced by higher-level processes (e.g. contextual, social, psychological); the disorder is not only dependent on lower-level phenomena (e.g. biology, chemistry, physics).(4)

The inadequacies of the biomedical model of illness have led, in the second half of the twentieth century, to the emergence of the biopsychosocial model of illness. The biopsychosocial model proposes to broaden the biomedical approach to include the psychosocial dimension with the aim to still care for patients from a disease standpoint and give psychological and social factors equal standing in the care process.(6) The biopsychosocial model of illness introduced the concept of top-down causality to the medical and healthcare world.(4) In top-down causality, the origin of an illness goes from causes at a higher level of organization to impact a lower level of organization (e.g. a headache caused by financial worries).(4)

The biopsychosocial model, despite its positive evaluations and success in some areas of healthcare (especially in rehabilitation), has not been fully integrated into everyday medical practice.(5) The lack of wider integration of the biopsychosocial model in the healthcare system is partly due to the lack of knowledge regarding the existence of the model. This lack of knowledge is widespread and includes healthcare staff (including managers), commissioners, funding agencies, and the public.(5) Another problem is that the model is too broad and provides little guidance to health professionals in finding relevant patient information.(6) The lack of inclusion of a method to identify factors that are ultimately responsible for a given condition is also an issue that impacts the integration of the model.(6) The patient ends up being again separated into different causal categories (biological, psychological, or social) that will be analyzed and treated in isolation from each other.(4) Furthermore, the biopsychosocial model of care almost exclusively considers cognition and behavior factors, and rarely gives attention to social context, culture, and power dynamics.(20)

The integration of the biopsychosocial model of care is a step in the right direction, albeit an insufficient one, since it ends up with the division of the biological, psychological, and social dimensions. Resistance to change from the biomedical model to the biopsychosocial model also impacted the wider acceptation of the new model. Any change in paradigm is likely to encounter barriers to its application. Global barriers to a change in paradigm, include elements from different domains:

- environmental contexts and resources (lack of time, cost, other colleagues, lack of expertise, patient preference)
- social influences (views from other colleagues)
- goals (incompatible with achieving other objectives)
- knowledge (lack of understanding of different models)
- beliefs about consequences (worse outcomes with a different model)
- beliefs about capabilities (level of confidence in applying a different model)
- behavioral regulation (clear plan on when to use a different model)
- intention (willingness to apply a new model).(21)(22)

Ontologically, changes in paradigm require changes in the basic underlying assumptions of the concept. A new model of care, such as the biopsychosocial model, will not result in the desired changes if it does not influence the practice and norms in place within the current model. The lack of a broader impact of the biopsychosocial model of illness, partly relies on the fact that the underlying reductionist and dualistic views of illness of the biomedical model have not changed with the advent of the new model. These views need to be updated to integrate the complexity and multi-causality characteristics of human conditions. Such a fundamental change in the core assumptions of healthcare should then result in changes in the organization, management, and financing of the system.(4)

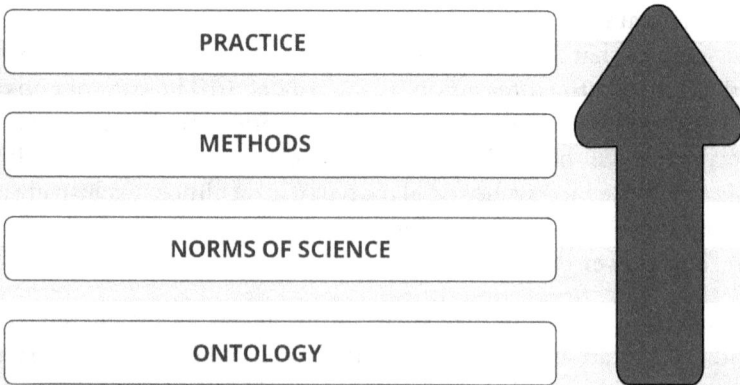

**Figure 1. A change in methods and practice must start from a change in ontology.** Reprinted under the terms of the Creative Commons Attribution 4.0 International License from Anjum RL, Copeland S, Rocca E. Rethinking Causality, Complexity and Evidence for the Unique Patient: A CauseHealth Resource for Healthcare Professionals and the Clinical Encounter.(4)

Ultimately, such foundational changes can lead to patient-centered care, guideline-concordant integrated care, improved patient experience and outcomes, and cost-effectiveness, which are the hallmarks of value-based care.(23)

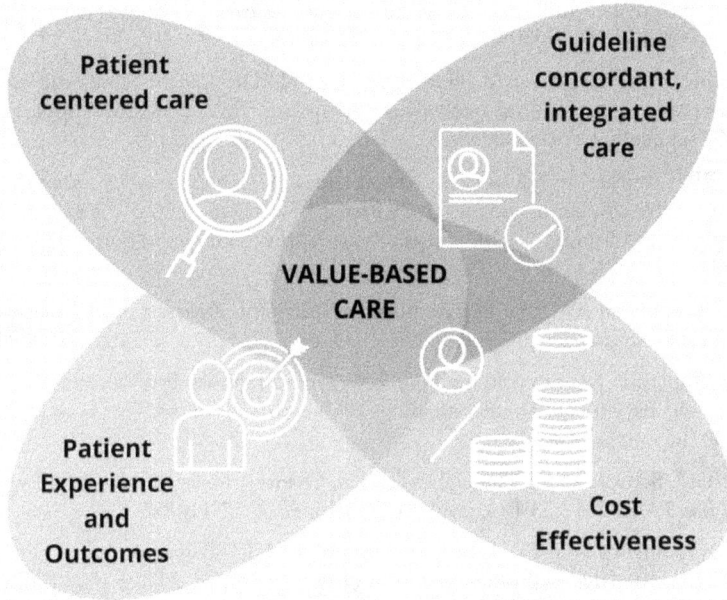

**Figure 2. The four components of value-based care.** Reprinted under the terms of the Creative Commons Attribution 4.0 International License from Cook CE, Denninger T, Lewis J, et al. Providing value-based care as a physiotherapist. Arch Physiother.(23)

# References

1. Briggs AM, Shiffman J, Shawar YR, et al. Global health policy in the 21st century: challenges and opportunities to arrest the global disability burden from musculoskeletal health conditions. *Best Pract Res Clin Rheumatol.* 2020;34(5):101549. doi:10.1016/j.berh.2020.101549

2. Foster NE, Anema JR, Cherkin D, et al. Prevention and treatment of low back pain: evidence, challenges, and promising directions. *Lancet.* 2018;391(10137):2368–2383. doi:10.1016/s0140-6736(18)30489-6

3. Buchbinder R, Underwood M, Hartvigsen J, et al. The Lancet Series call to action to reduce low value care for low back pain: an update. *Pain.* 2020;161(Suppl 1):S57–S64. doi:10.1097/j.pain.0000000000001869

4. Anjum RL, Copeland S, Rocca E. *Rethinking Causality, Complexity and Evidence for the Unique Patient: A CauseHealth Resource for Healthcare Professionals and the Clinical Encounter.* New York, NY: Springer Publishing; 2020. https://www.springer.com/gp/book/9783030412388. Accessed Jan 15, 2021.

5. Wade DT, Halligan PW. The biopsychosocial model of illness: a model whose time has come. *Clinical Rehabilitation.* 2017;31(8):995–1004. doi:10.1177/0269215517709890

6. Farre A, Rapley T. The new old (and old new) medical model: four decades navigating the biomedical and psychosocial understandings of health and illness. *Healthcare.* 2017;5(4):88. doi:10.3390/healthcare5040088

7. Brodersen J, Schwartz LM, Heneghan C, et al. Overdiagnosis: what it is and what it isn't. *BMJ Evid Based Med.* 2018;23:1–3. doi:10.1136/ebmed-2017-110886

8. Lee CS, Goldhaber NH, Davis SM, et al. Shoulder MRI in asymptomatic elite volleyball athletes shows extensive pathology. *Jt Disord Orthop Sport Med.* 2020;5:10–14. doi:10.1136/jisakos-2019-000304

9. Lähdeoja T, Karjalainen T, Jokihaara J, et al. Subacromial decompression surgery for adults with shoulder pain: a systematic review with meta-analysis. *Br J Sport Med.* 2020;54(11):665–673. doi:10.1136/bjsports-2018-100486

10. Harris IA, Sidhu V, Mittal R, et al. Surgery for chronic musculoskeletal pain: the question of evidence. *Pain.* 2020;161(Suppl 1):S95–S103. doi:10.1097/j.pain.0000000000001881

11. Kemp JL, Østerås N, Mathiessen A, et al. Relationship between cam morphology, hip symptoms, and hip osteoarthritis: the Musculoskeletal pain in Ullersaker STudy (MUST) cohort. *HIP Int.* 2020. doi:10.1177/1120700020943853

12. van Klij P, Ginai AZ, Heijboer MP, et al. The relationship between cam morphology and hip and groin symptoms and signs in young male football players. *Scand J Med Sci Sports.* 2020;30(7):1221–1231. doi:10.1111/sms.13660

13. Blankenstein T, Grainger A, Dube B, et al. MRI hip findings in asymptomatic professional rugby players, ballet dancers, and age-matched controls. *Clin Radiol.* 2020;75(2):116–122. doi:10.1016/j.crad.2019.08.024

14. Culvenor AG, Øiestad BE, Hart HF, et al. Prevalence of knee osteoarthritis features on magnetic resonance imaging in asymptomatic uninjured adults: a systematic review and meta-analysis. *Br J Sports Med.* 2019;53(20):1268–1278. doi:10.1136/bjsports-2018-09925

15. Bacon K, LaValley MP, Jafarzadeh SR, et al. Does cartilage loss cause pain in osteoarthritis and if so, how much? *Ann Rheum Dis*. 2020;79(8):1105–1110. doi:10.1136/annrheumdis-2020-217363

16. Son KM, Hong JI, Kim D-H, et al. Absence of pain in subjects with advanced radiographic knee osteoarthritis. *BMC Musculoskelet Disord*. 2020;21:1–9. doi:10.1186/s12891-020-03647-x

17. Simo S, Liisa K, Katariina L, et al. Disc degeneration of young low back pain patients. *Spine (Phila Pa 1976)*. 2020;45(19):1341–1347. doi:10.1097/brs.0000000000003548

18. Udby PM, Ohrt-Nissen S, Bendix T, et al. The Association of MRI findings and long-term disability in patients with chronic low back pain. *SAGE Open Med*. 2020. doi:10.1177/2192568220921391

19. Daimon K, Fujiwara H, Nishiwaki Y, et al. A 20-year prospective longitudinal study of degeneration of the cervical spine in a volunteer cohort assessed using MRI. *J Bone Jt Surg*. 2018;100(10):843–849. doi:10.2106/jbjs.17.01347

20. Mescouto K, Olson RE, Hodges PW, et al. A critical review of the biopsychosocial model of low back pain care: time for a new approach? *Disabil Rehabil*. 2020;1–15. doi:10.1080/09638288.2020.1851783

21. AL Zoubi FM, French SD, Patey AM, et al. Professional barriers and facilitators to using stratified care approaches for managing non-specific low back pain: a qualitative study with Canadian physiotherapists and chiropractors. *Chiropr Man Therap*. 2019;27:68. doi:10.1186/s12998-019-0286-3

22. Lewis J, O'Sullivan P, O'Sullivan P. Is it time to reframe how we care for people with non-traumatic musculoskeletal pain? *BR J Sports Med*. 2018;1543–1544. doi:10.1136/bjsports-2018-099198

23. Cook CE, Denninger T, Lewis J, et al. Providing value-based care as a physiotherapist. *Arch Physiother*. 2021;11:12. doi:10.1186/s40945-021-00107-0

# Dispositionalism Model

Both the biomedical and biopsychosocial models of care view the person as a whole, who is best understood by separately assessing and treating individual parts (the liver, the heart, the lungs, etc. for the biomedical model; the biology, the psychology, and the social for the biopsychosocial model). The individual parts exist and function for themselves and do not, nor are they influenced by, the other parts. (This can be likened to parts of a car engine that form a functional unit, but can be separated into individual parts that function by themselves.) In order to truly adopt a whole-person approach, a foundational change in the understanding of complexity is required.[1]

Complexity in biological systems (and other systems) is more than merely putting together individual parts to build a whole (e.g. constructing a car engine). Another view of complexity is to see complex wholes consisting of parts that interact with each other in a way that also influences and alters the parts themselves in the process.[1] The interaction of the parts within that whole gives identity to each part[1] as well as to the whole. The functional role of each part is defined by its place and interaction as part of that particular whole.[1],[2] Outside of the whole, the parts would not be that particular part with those particular dispositions.[1]

Dispositions, also described as abilities, capacities, or causal powers, refer to what something can do.[1],[2],[3] Dispositions are intrinsic properties belonging to an individual or entity that can exist unmanifested.[1],[3] A crystal glass is fragile and can be broken. A sharp blade can cut. A virus can make a healthy person sick. Dispositions exist as such, even if unmanifested, and can influence an individual or entity differently at different times and under different circumstances. A crystal glass will break if it falls from a certain height, with a certain force, onto a hard enough surface. Dispositions might not be observable until they manifest themselves.[1],[3] Typically, when dispositions manifest themselves, causality happens.[1] For example, every individual has the disposition to develop cancer. Cancer cells are neutralized on a daily basis by the immune system, but under certain circumstances, these cancer cells might become unchecked and grow into a disease. Consequently, the dispositional property is a cause, and the manifestation is an effect.(1)

The manifestation of a disorder (e.g. a symptom), is rarely associated with one single disposition, but with a set of dispositions.(2) Two or more dispositions will interact with each other and produce a causality they could not do in isolation.(2),(4) Manifestations are produced by the interaction of multiple dispositions, therefore, different contexts will manifest themselves differently. This means that, from a dispositionalist perspective, all causality is complex because it requires the interaction of one or more sets of dispositions that need to be considered in the context of the interaction. Everything that contributes to the manifestation is viewed as a cause. Thus, dispositions are useful for understanding the illness experience, making the correct diagnosis, and selecting the appropriate treatment strategy.(1) A headache can be caused by stress, or by a tumor in the brain. Knowing and understanding not only the individual dispositions, but also the cultural, societal, and contextual dispositions at play for each patient, will help determine the causes of the disorder, the pain experienced by the patient, and the treatment strategy most likely to result in desired outcomes.

In dispositionalism, a complex "whole" can never be completely understood by observing its "parts" in isolation.(1) The interaction between the parts, and their impact on the whole, is as important for causality as the individual parts themselves.(1) The whole is the result of a continuous and complex interaction among the parts, during which time the parts influence each other and evolve. The whole is, therefore, more than the sum of its parts. (1) As the parts evolve due to their interactions, a whole with new properties and dispositions will emerge.

In order to understand and care for living beings, complex interactions need to be understood. A whole person is made up of parts (e.g. a liver, a heart, a brain). There is important and meaningful knowledge to gain from studying each part, however, the identity of every single part lies in its interactions with other parts — the person's context, their history, and their lived experience. (1) Clinicians, therefore, need to view health and illness as a manifestation of physiological and biochemical processes, and, equally important, as a manifestation of internal, external, and contextual causes. This requires clinicians to start looking at the person from the higher level of complexity — the whole — which, in turn, enables them to focus on interactions between context, lived experience, and physical body parts.(1) Therefore, a disposition-based care model is better suited to address the complexities of patients suffering from musculoskeletal disorders. A contemporary, patient-centered, disposition-based model of care, offers solutions to practitioners with evidence-based treatment for MSK conditions.(5)

The dispositionalism model can be illustrated using vectors. The vectors represent the dispositions that are present at a particular time, for a particular person, and contribute to that person's condition.(1) This means the length and direction of the vectors, as well as the type of disposition represented by the vectors, will vary from one individual to another.(1) The reason for this is that the vectors represent the singularism of causal dispositionalism — that causality happens in a unique particular context.(1) Furthermore, vectors show two important characteristics of dispositions — their degree of strength and their direction.(1) All dispositions - both the ones that tend toward, and the ones that tend away from, a manifestation (i.e. a symptom) - need to be included. The integration of all the vectors will yield a resultant vector (R) that will show the tendency toward the manifestation, as shown in the following diagram.

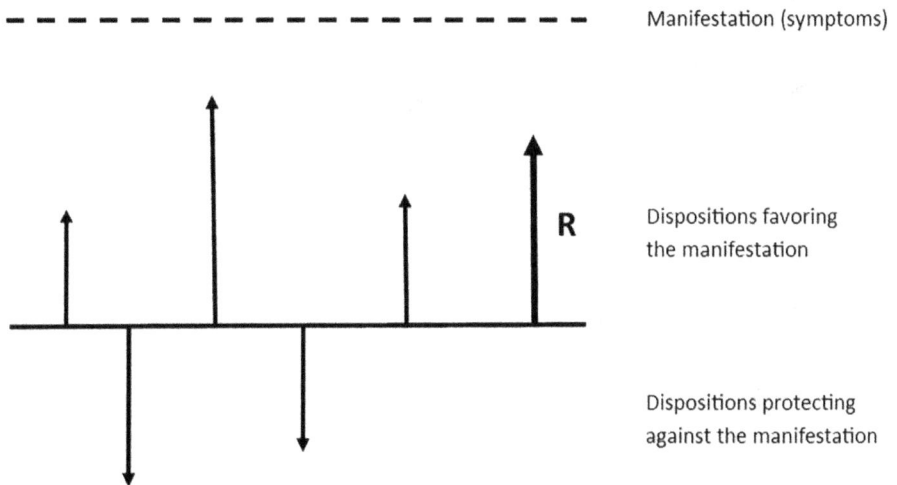

**Figure 3. The vector model of causality.** The vectors demonstrate some central features of causality — different types of causal interference, different degrees of tendency, threshold effects, and tipping points — in addition to causal complexity and causal sensitivity.(1) R=resultant vector.

People affected by MSK disorders, present with a multitude of factors influencing their disorder's manifestations. The dispositionalism model can help both patients and clinicians uncover and understand these dispositions, and, in turn, better understand what leads to the clinical picture. The vector model helps with the visualization of the dispositions at play and provides the basis for discussion about the dispositions and their interactions. The discussion that ensues will get patients actively involved in the delivery of care, which will foster trust, respect, and therapeutic alliance. Management strategies can then be aimed at the dispositions having the most impact on a patient's presentation, leading to individualized, patient-centered care.

# References

1. Anjum RL, Copeland S, Rocca E. *Rethinking Causality, Complexity and Evidence for the Unique Patient: A CauseHealth Resource for Healthcare Professionals and the Clinical Encounter.* New York, NY: Springer Publishing; 2020. https://www.springer.com/gp/book/9783030412388. Accessed Jan 21, 2021.

2. Anjum RL, Mumford S. Dispositionalism: a dynamic theory of causation. OUP. 2018. doi: 10.1093/oso/9780198779636.003.0003

3. Rocca E, Anjum RL. Causal evidence and dispositions in medicine and public health. *Int J Environ Res Public Health.* 2020;17(6):1–18. doi:10.3390/ijerph17061813

4. Baltimore JA. Dispositionalism, causation, and the interaction gap. *Erkenn.* 2020;1–16. doi:10.1007/s10670-019-00213-3

5. Kerry R, Low M, O'Sullivan P. Person-centered clinical reasoning and evidence-based healthcare. *EJPCH.* 2020;8(2). doi:10.5750/ejpch.v8i2.1845

# Predictive Processing

—◯✕◯—

Explanations of illness causality include top-down or bottom-up processes (see chapter: Change in Paradigm). Bottom-up explanations look for causes of disorders at the physical level, while top-down explanations emphasize higher-level causes of illness, such as contextual, psychological, or social. (1) Top-down and bottom-up processes happen together synchronously, whereby one influences the other. Causality depends on the reciprocal hierarchical organization of information processing in the brain and undergoes predictive processing.

The brain has long been considered a passive system awaiting sensory input to perceive reality and reacting upon the information it receives.(2),(3),(4) Newer neuroscientific research shows quite the contrary; the brain actively makes predictions as to the causes and the nature of incoming sensory signals and compares these predictions to the actual input.(5),(6),(7),(8),(9) Errors in predictions are then used to update the brain models to minimize discrepancies.(5),(6),(7),(8),(9) This process allows the brain to encode information about the sources of sensory signals and drive future predictions. (2),(5),(6),(7),(8),(9)

An example of predictions and prediction errors in the brain is the culinary trompe l'oeil (to deceive the eye). A fried egg is on a plate. The brain predicts, based on experience, the taste the egg is expected to have. Upon tasting, the egg tastes like an apricot cheesecake. The discrepancy between the sensory input and the prediction — the prediction error — surprises the brain, makes the brain double-check what the food is, and updates its expectation for the next bite. This next bite is less surprising as the brain updated its prediction to minimize the prediction error. Essentially, the brain is a prediction machine. This process is known as predictive processing.

Predictive processing is necessary because, during any kind of perceptive experience, humans can rely only on previous experiences and sensory information.(10) The sensory information an individual can access is, however, almost always ambiguous, incomplete, or noisy.(10) Therefore, the world is perceived by statistically estimating the most likely properties of the world, on the basis of noisy information.(10)

Predictive processing says that perception results from the brain inferring the most likely causes and the nature of its sensory inputs by minimizing the difference between the actual sensory signals and the signals expected on the basis of continuously updated predictive models.(3),(5),(6),(7),(8) ,(11),(12),(13),(14),(15),(16),(17) Predictive processing emphasizes the importance of hierarchical systems which develop, refine, and deploy these predictions.(2),(6),(7),(8),(9) Predictions are compared against the actual sensory input at multiple levels of cortical hierarchy. Higher-level cortical hierarchies carry top-down predictions to lower hierarchical levels.(5),(6),(7),(8),(9) Lower-level cortical hierarchies carry bottom-up prediction errors to higher cortical levels.(5),(6),(7),(8),(9) This means the brain can generate a representation of the causes and the nature of sensory input, by relying only on signals to which it has direct access — predictions and prediction errors.(5),(6),(7),(8),(9)

The predictive brain model is a bidirectional hierarchical cascade.(6),(7),(8),(9) Multiple levels of processing in multiple cortical areas of the brain are involved in predictive processing, giving the model its cascading properties.(6),(7),(8),(9) The model is hierarchical because it relies on higher and lower levels of processing.(6),(7)(8)(9) The lower levels process simple data, such as sensory stimuli, motor commands, and affective signals. Higher levels process categorizations such as object recognition, emotion classification, and action selection. The highest levels process mental states such as emotional experience, goal setting, planning, reasoning, and mental imagery. Bidirectionality describes the continuous propagation of signals in both upward and downward directions.(6),(7),(8),(9) Sensory information and prediction errors are carried up the chain from lower levels to higher levels of processing and, inversely, predictions and motor commands are carried down from higher levels to lower levels.

Prediction errors can be minimized by updating parameters of the predictive models to fit incoming data, or by performing actions to change sensory data to fit or test the models.(5),(4) Model updating is optimized by giving preference to sensory data that is expected to carry more information.(5),(4) This attention to sensory data relies on the expected precision of the information being perceived. The precision of the prediction errors determines the attention the information will be given in the hierarchical cascade. Precision is a measure of the brain's trust in the information it receives. Prediction errors with a low level of precision will carry less weight and, therefore, be given less attention than prediction errors with a high level of precision. For example, visual information in a dark, foggy setting is not as reliable as information on a clear, sunny day. Therefore, the visual information gained on the dark, foggy day will not carry a high level of expected precision, and the prediction errors associated with that visual information will not be given much attention in the hierarchical processing. Information that elicits a strong reaction will also be given more attention and has increased potential to update the model. Pain catastrophizing is an example of a strong emotional reaction to a nociceptive input, that has the potential to change the brain's prediction about the pain experience, and increase the likelihood of the development of chronic pain (see chapter: Pain Catastrophizing). In most cases, these processes run continuously and simultaneously, providing a deep continuity between perception and action,(5) thus allowing the body to adapt and learn from new contexts and responses.

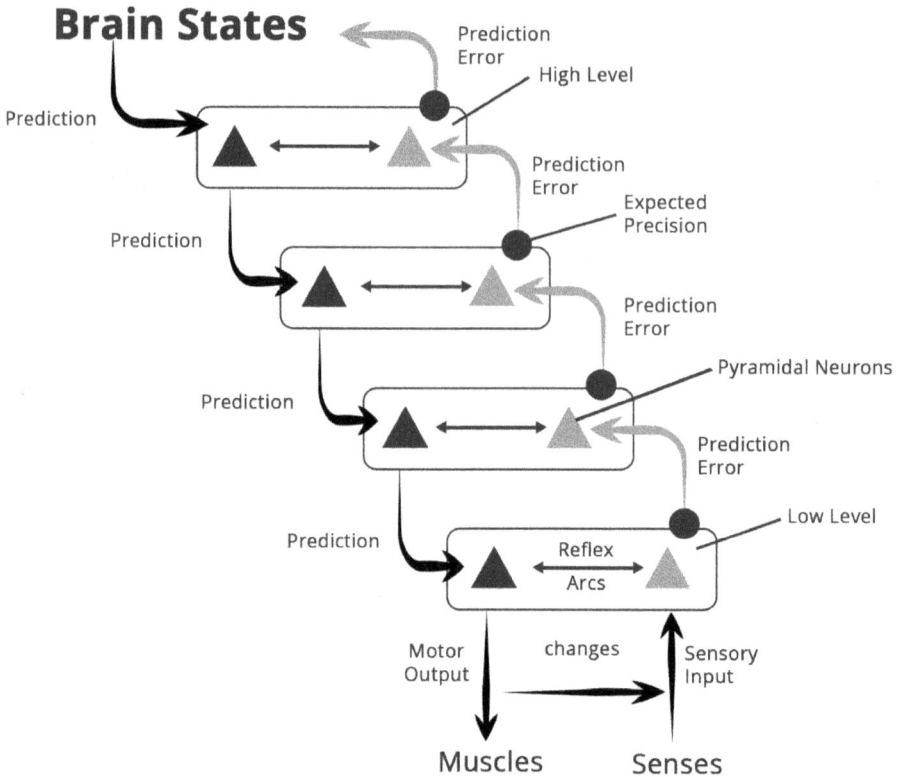

**Figure 4. Schematic depiction of a bidirectional hierarchical cascade.** Adapted with permission from author from https://www.mindcoolness.com/blog/bayesian-brain-predictive-processing.

Nociception is required, but is not sufficient to elicit the perception of pain. The peripheral nociceptive information needs to reach higher cortical centers and is submitted, on its way, to influences from the spinal cord, the brainstem, the thalamus, and the limbic system before reaching the cortex. Therefore, pain perception is also the result of a probability function based on incomplete or noisy information(10) and is submitted to predictive processing.(4) The brain makes inferences based on incomplete information during the experience of pain, just as it does during other sensory input. (10) The processing of pain is, therefore, also subjected to predictions and prediction errors that can be minimized or amplified by perceptions and actions, and is subjected to cortical hierarchical organization.(4) Nociceptive and non-nociceptive information is integrated with hierarchical predictive processing models to calculate the experience that would most benefit the immediate objective of the individual. Any resulting credible indication of threat to body tissue can increase pain perception, while any resulting credible indication of safety to body tissue can decrease pain perception.(10)

Individual beliefs and expectations can dramatically influence the predictions a person makes, and can be a source of bias of incoming sensory data. (2) A wide range of cognitive and psychological phenomena and biases, can be conceptualized in the predictive processing model. For example, placebo analgesia and the nocebo effect result from top-down expectations modulating bottom-up sensory signals in a hierarchical predictive processing framework.(2) Likewise, kinesiophobia results from a higher-level prediction or belief that movement is going to be painful or harmful, and modulates the lower-level patient's behavior (i.e. patient not performing certain movements or activities), to match the expected outcome. Psychological factors (or higher-level cognition), such as catastrophizing, can increase the perceived threat to body tissue and modulate incoming sensory signals (or lower-level signals) (i.e. augmentation of nociceptive signals), to increase pain perception in order to diminish the discrepancy between the predicted and actual perception.

Predictive processing helps clinicians to better understand the neurophysiological processes involved in pain processing and perception. That knowledge can be used to educate patients about dispositions at play in their MSK disorders, and can inform shared decision-making about management strategies. The good news is that the plasticity of the brain, as described in the predictive processing framework, can be used therapeutically to update the prediction models of the brain, by using targeted sensory input that elicits clinically meaningful responses, that will be carried up the cascade to higher cortical centers, potentially changing a patient's pain cognition and behavior.

# References

1. Anjum RL, Copeland S, Rocca E. *Rethinking Causality, Complexity and Evidence for the Unique Patient: A CauseHealth Resource for Healthcare Professionals and the Clinical Encounter.* New York, NY: Springer Publishing; 2020. https://www.springer.com/gp/book/9783030412388. Accessed Jan 21, 2021.

2. Bissell DA, Ziadni MS, Sturgeon JA. Perceived injustice in chronic pain: an examination through the lens of predictive processing. *Pain Manag.* 2018;8(2):129–138. doi:10.2217/pmt-2017-0051

3. Thornton C. Predictive processing simplified: The infotropic machine. *Brain Cogn.* 2017;112:13–24. doi:10.1016/j.bandc.2016.03.004

4. Barrett LF, Simmons WK. Interoceptive predictions in the brain. *Nat Rev Neurosci.* 2015;16(7):419–29. doi:10.1038/nrn3950

5. Seth AK. The cybernetic Bayesian brain from interoceptive inference to sensorimotor contingencies. *Open MIND.* 2015:1-24. doi:10.15502/9783958570108

6. Rao RP, Ballard DH. Predictive coding in the visual cortex: A functional interpretation of some extra-classical receptive-field effects. *Nat Neurosci.* 1999;2:79–87. doi:10.1038/4580

7. Lee TS, Mumford D. Hierarchical Bayesian inference in the visual cortex. *J Opt Soc Am A Opt Image Sci Vis.* 2003;20(7):1434–1448. doi:10.1364/josaa.20.001434

8. Friston K. A theory of cortical responses. *Philos Trans R Soc Lond B Biol Sci.* 2005;360(1456):815–836. doi:10.1098/rstb.2005.1622

9. Clark A. Whatever next? Predictive brains, situated agents, and the future of cognitive science. *Behav Brain Sci.* 2013;36(3):181–204. doi:10.1017/s0140525x12000477

10. Tabor A, Thacker MA, Moseley GL, et al. Pain: a statistical account. *PLOS Comput Biol.* 2017;13:e1005142. doi:10.1371/journal.pcbi.1005142

11. Spratling MW. Predictive coding as a model of biased competition in visual attention. *Vision Res.* 2008;48(12):1391–1408. doi:10.1016/j.visres.2008.03.009

12. Knill DC, Pouget A. The Bayesian brain: the role of uncertainty in neural coding and computation. *Trends Neurosci.* 2004;27(12):712-719. doi:10.1016/j.tins.2004.10.007

13. Jehee JF, Ballard DH. Predictive feedback can account for biphasic responses in the lateral geniculate nucleus. *PLoS Comput Biol.* 2009;5(5):e1000373. doi:10.1371/journal.pcbi.1000373

14. Huang Y, Rao RP. Predictive coding. *Wiley Interdiscip Rev Cogn Sci.* 2011;2(5):580-593. doi:10.1002/wcs.142

15. Friston K. The free-energy principle: a unified brain theory? *Nat Rev Neurosci.* 2010;11(2):127-138. doi:10.1038/nrn2787

16. Clark A. *Surfing Uncertainty: Prediction, Action, and the Embodied Mind.* New York, NY: Oxford University Press; 2016. https://oxford.universitypressscholarship.com/view/10.1093/acprof:oso/9780190217013.001.0001/acprof-9780190217013. Accessed Jan 10, 2021.

17. Brown H, Friston K, Bestmann S. Active inference, attention, and motor preparation. *Front Psychol.* 2011;2:218. doi:10.3389/fpsyg.2011.00218

# The Common Sense Model

People experiencing pain try to make sense of their experience to gain control of the pain experience and its impact on their life. The inability to control pain and its impact, creates a set of negative affective responses that influences pain response and behavior, elicits a fear response, and can maintain a painful state as described in the fear-avoidance model.(1),(2)

The fear-avoidance model (see chapter: Pain Catastrophizing) is a well-known example of the Common Sense Model (CSM). The fear-avoidance model captures one particular type of sense-making, namely catastrophizing, and identifies the two main factors that play a role — negative affect and threatening illness information.(1)

The sense-making process of people experiencing pain-related fear is far more encompassing than what is described in the fear-avoidance model and includes other constructs that influence behavior in MSK conditions. (1) The CSM accounts for this broader, sense-making process and includes multiple influencing factors (i.e. outcome expectancies, self-efficacy, goals, sociostructural factors, emotional or stress constructs, and symptom-related control) and can help in understanding the fear-avoidance cycle.(1)

The CSM states that when a symptom is experienced, the person tries to make sense of the symptom by forming a cognitive representation.(1),(2),(3),(4) This representation is based on a set of beliefs that include:

1. the identity of the symptom (e.g. a herniated disc)

2. the cause of the symptom (e.g. heavy lifting in a bad position)

3. the consequences of the symptom (e.g. physical incapacity)

4. the controllability of the symptom (e.g. activity avoidance)

5. the timeline of the symptom (e.g. will never go away).(1),(2),(3),(4)

These beliefs can be formed, as in the fear-avoidance model, either by previous direct experiences of the symptom, vicarious experiences observing others with similar symptoms, or information learned about the symptom from sources such as the media and clinicians.(2),(3) Beliefs about a symptom can, therefore, be formed before actually directly experiencing the symptom and will influence the representation of the symptom. The inability to make sense of a symptom will elicit a fear response.(1),(2)

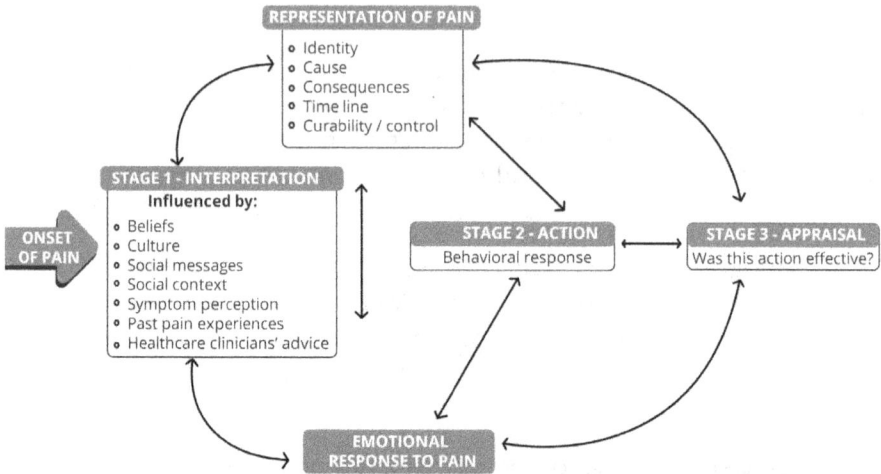

Figure 5. **Common Sense Model framework.** Reprinted with permission from publisher from Caneiro JP, Bunzli S, O'Sullivan P. Beliefs about the body and pain: the critical role in musculoskeletal pain management. Brazilian J Phys Ther.(2)

The representation of the symptom informs what actions will be undertaken to deal with the symptom; a process known as problem-solving behavior. (1),(2) The emotional response to the symptom (emotion-directed coping) is also influenced by the representation of the symptom. Problem-solving behavior and emotion-directed coping undergo predictive processing (see chapter: Predictive Processing). The highest levels of brain processing (goal setting, planning, and reasoning) will, for example, predict the expected outcome of a behavior on the symptom, based on the representation of the symptom (e.g. less pain by avoidance behavior), and will give information to the next lower level of processing to put the plan in motion. That lower level of processing will select an action or actions (e.g. not bending forward) that will most likely result in the predicted outcome. The information is then passed down to the lowest level of processing that will initiate motor commands to physically complete the task. Sensory and affective information from the lowest levels of processing will then be sent upward to the higher and highest levels of processing, which will compare the incoming information to the initial prediction. If the outcome of the behavior matches the prediction, the representation of the symptom will be perceived as accurate and useful and will be reinforced. On the contrary, if the outcome of the behavior does not match the brain's prediction (prediction error), the representation of the symptom will be perceived as ineffective and will be updated with the new information and experience. The same processes are found in emotion-directed coping. Hence, due to the continuous interaction between cognition, behavior, and context, the representation of symptoms is dynamic and ever-evolving.

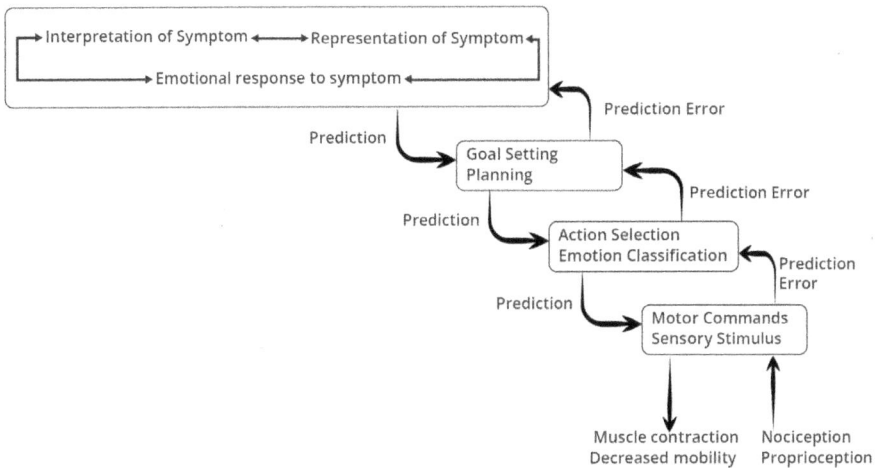

**Figure 6. Common Sense Model bidirectional hierarchical cascade.**

Better knowledge and integration of the broader, sense-making process and its elements by the clinician leads to a better understanding of a patient's dispositions at play in the clinical presentation. This can be used to foster the therapeutic alliance and the development of a collaborative management plan, thereby improving treatment outcomes. The evolving nature of the representation of the symptom can lead to avoidance behavior and disability but it also offers an entry gate to management interventions (e.g. exposure treatments).

# References

1. Bunzli S, Smith A, Schütze R, et al. Making sense of low back pain and pain-related fear. *J Orthop Sport Phys Ther*. 2017;47(9):628–636. doi:10.2519/jospt.2017.7434

2. Caneiro JP, Bunzli S, O'Sullivan P. Beliefs about the body and pain: the critical role in musculoskeletal pain management. *Brazilian J Phys Ther*. 2021;25(1):17–29. doi:10.1016/j.bjpt.2020.06.003

3. Leventhal H, Diefenbach M, Leventhal EA. Illness cognition: using common sense to understand treatment adherence and affect cognition interactions. *Cognit Ther Res*. 1992;16(2):143–163. doi:10.1007/bf01173486

4. Leventhal H, Phillips LA, Burns E. The common-sense model of self-regulation (CSM): a dynamic framework for understanding illness self-management. *J Behav Med*. 2016;39(6):935–946. doi:10.1007/s10865-016-9782-2

# The Context

# Clinical Encounter

————∞————

The clinical encounter describes the interaction between the patient and the clinician, during which transactions between patients and health professionals take place,(1) that are fundamental to clinical care.(2) It is the human element of the therapeutic relationship that is at the center of health care delivery. The clinical encounter is the point at which patients and clinicians get to know each other, and decisions about diagnosis and treatments are made.(1)

Patients place high value on clinical encounters and see them as central to their health; and clinical encounters affect health outcomes.(1) Positive clinical encounters are associated with higher patient satisfaction, mutual trust, treatment adherence, and improved clinical outcomes.(2),(3) On the other hand, suboptimal interactions may discourage care-seeking and propagate miscommunication, clinician burnout, and patient distrust.(2)

In turn, positive clinical encounters foster patient-centered collaborative care which is of central importance for patient management. Patient-centered care has been associated with higher patient satisfaction, better patient adherence, better patient outcomes (such as a reduction in concern and discomfort), better self-reported health, improved physiological status, and lower costs of care.(4)

Clinical encounters never happen in a vacuum but, rather, in a complex set of contextual factors that can be viewed as the "atmosphere around the treatment"(5) or "contextual healing".(6),(7) Contextual factors independently influence the clinical encounter and treatment outcomes, and can be:

- internal (dispositions of the patient)
- external (clinical environment, characteristics of the treatment, clinician's dispositions)
- relational (patient-physician relationship — verbal information, therapeutic alliance).(7),(8),(9),(10)

Patient-physician relationships and treatment outcomes are associated with brain-behavioral mechanisms.(2) Neural mechanisms underpinning the patient-clinician interaction include nonverbal behavioral mirroring and brain-to-brain concordance in circuitry, implicated in theory of mind and social mirroring.(2) Extensive dynamic coupling of these brain nodes with a partner's brain activity, modulates the treatment outcome in patient-clinician partners who have a pre-established clinical rapport.(2) These findings underscore the impotence of a positive clinical encounter to improve clinical outcomes (see Appendix A).

The aim of this book is to discuss contextual factors and the mechanisms at play during the management of MSK disorders. Knowledge and understanding of these factors can help clinicians to better understand their patients, themselves, and the interactions taking place during patient-clinician exchanges. The awareness of these dispositions can help physicians improve themselves and the care they deliver to patients, leading to a true patient-centered collaborative therapeutic alliance. Physician-patient collaboration is, in turn, associated with better patient adherence and outcomes,(1),(11) and care, delivered in a positive context, produces better outcomes.(7)

# References

1. Dieppe P, Rafferty A, Kitson A. The clinical encounter - the focal point of patient-centred care. *Health Expect.* 2002;5(4):279. doi:10.1046/j.1369-6513.2002.00198.x

2. Ellingsen D-M, Isenburg K, Jung C, et al. Dynamic brain-to-brain concordance and behavioral mirroring as a mechanism of the patient-clinician interaction. *Sci Adv.* 2020;6(43):eabc1304. doi:10.1126/sciadv.abc1304

3. Griffin AR, Moloney M, Leaver A, et al. Experiences of responsiveness to exercise in people with chronic whiplash: a qualitative study. *Musculoskelet Sci Pract.* 2021;54:102380. doi:10.1016/j.msksp.2021.102380

4. Ryan BL, Brown JB, Tremblay PF, et al. Measuring patients' perceptions of health care encounters: examining the factor structure of the revised patient perception of patient-centeredness (PPPC-R) questionnaire. *J Patient-Cent Res Rev.* 2019;6(3):192–202. doi:10.17294/2330-0698.1696

5. Balint M. The doctor, his patient, and the illness. *Lancet.* 1955;265(6866):683–688. doi:10.1016/S0140-6736(55)91061-8

6. Miller FG, Kaptchuk TJ. The power of context: reconceptualizing the placebo effect. *JR Soc Med.* 2008;101(5):222–225. doi:10.1258/jrsm.2008.070466

7. Rossettini G, Carlino E, Testa M. Clinical relevance of contextual factors as triggers of placebo and nocebo effects in musculoskeletal pain. *BMC Musculoskelet Disord.* 2018;19:27. doi:10.1186/s12891-018-1943-8

8. Carlino E, Benedetti F. Different contexts, different pains, different experiences. *Neuroscience.* 2016;338:19-26. doi:10.1016/j.neuroscience.2016.01.053

9. Benedetti F. Placebo and the new physiology of the doctor-patient relationship. *Physiol Rev.* 2013:93(3):1207-1246. doi:10.1152/physrev.00043.2012

10. Perfitt JS, Plunkett N, Jones S. Placebo effect in the management of chronic pain. *BJA Educ.* 2020;20(11):382-387. doi:10.1016/j.bjae.2020.07.002

11. Arbuthnott A, Sharpe D. The effect of physician-patient collaboration on patient adherence in non-psychiatric medicine. *Patient Educ Couns.* 2009;77:60–67. doi:10.1016/j.pec.2009.03.022

# Contextual Dispositions

Cognitive, emotional, and sensory processes that modulate pain, arise from the context surrounding the pain experience.(1),(2) A positive and rewarding context can lead to pain relief and clinical improvement.(1),(2) A negative context can exacerbate pain and worsen clinical outcomes.(1),(2) Contextual factors are relevant to the clinician-patient relationship, and to treatment success, and should not be underrated.(3),(4),(5)

The context is made up of anything surrounding the patient during the pain experience and patient care. Contextual dispositions that affect therapeutic outcomes include external sensory and social stimuli, such as:

- the characteristics of the treatment — color and shape of a pill
- the healthcare setting — clinical environment and room layout
- the medical equipment — machines, needles, tables
- the clinician's characteristics — cognitive and affective communication, attitudes, behaviors (such as empathy, treatment and illness beliefs), status, sex, culture (see chapters in section: The Clinician)
- administration ritual.(1),(3),(4)

Internal variables, such as a patient's psychological and personal traits, motivations, optimism, treatment and illness beliefs, trust, and cognitive and affective histories (anxiety/fear), also play a key role (see chapters in section: The Patient).(1),(3),(4) The interaction of the external and internal variables, the patient-clinician relationship (i.e. suggestions, reassurance, compassion, and therapeutic alliance) is also a contextual factor of central importance. (3) The consideration of all these factors is required to genuinely care for patients, not only to treat them.

A positive context relies on two main mechanisms — positive expectations and classical conditioning.(1),(4),(6),(7) Expectations rely on prior experience and social learning, while conditioning depends on a learned response to a specific stimulus.(4) In the first mechanism, positive contextual elements that promote benefits can reduce fear and activate reward mechanisms.(1),(6) The activation of reward mechanisms plays a key role in the activation of the behavioral activation system (BAS), that is linked to approach behaviors and a greater positive function, despite pain (see chapter: Pain Catastrophizing). The functionality and efficiency of the reward system are dependent on the responsiveness of the dopaminergic system and the nucleus accumbens. (1),(5),(6) Dopamine and the nucleus accumbens are also involved in neurobiological pathways for pain and depression, partly explaining their comorbidity (see chapter: Depression). Prosocial hormones, like oxytocin and vasopressin, also play a role in contextual analgesia by modulating social factors, such as trust.(1),(5) Oxytocin promotes intimacy and social interaction, and is involved in the modulation effects of verbal support on pain between companions (see chapter: Social Determinants of Health).

The second mechanism involves repeated associations between external cues and intervention, with positive outcomes that can lead to a conditioned response, whereby the external cues will elicit a response without the actual intervention (e.g. color, shape, and taste of an analgesic pill, with or without the active ingredient).(1)

A negative context, such as verbal suggestions of pain increase or a negative warning promoted by clinicians, family, friends, or mass media, may negatively impact perceived symptoms.(1) These preformed beliefs about diagnoses and prognoses can negatively impact symptoms and treatment outcomes (see chapter: The Common Sense Model). The way of communicating diagnoses and associated prognoses that can be perceived as negative by patients can lead to an amplification of pain, and negatively affect a patient's emotions (e.g. a crumbled spine causing low back pain). Distrust towards clinicians and therapies, influenced by the quality of the patient-clinician relationship, can also potentiate symptoms.

Pain modulation involving verbal suggestions activates a descending pain modulating network.(1) The patterns of brain activation in that descending pathway mostly involve three key brain areas: the prefrontal cortex, the anterior cingulate cortex, and the periaqueductal gray.(1),(2),(4),(5),(6),(8) The same brain areas are involved in the reciprocal modulation of pain and depression, and are associated with increased nociception, heightened attention to pain, and promotion of negative affect in both conditions (see chapter: Depression).

**Contextual factors**

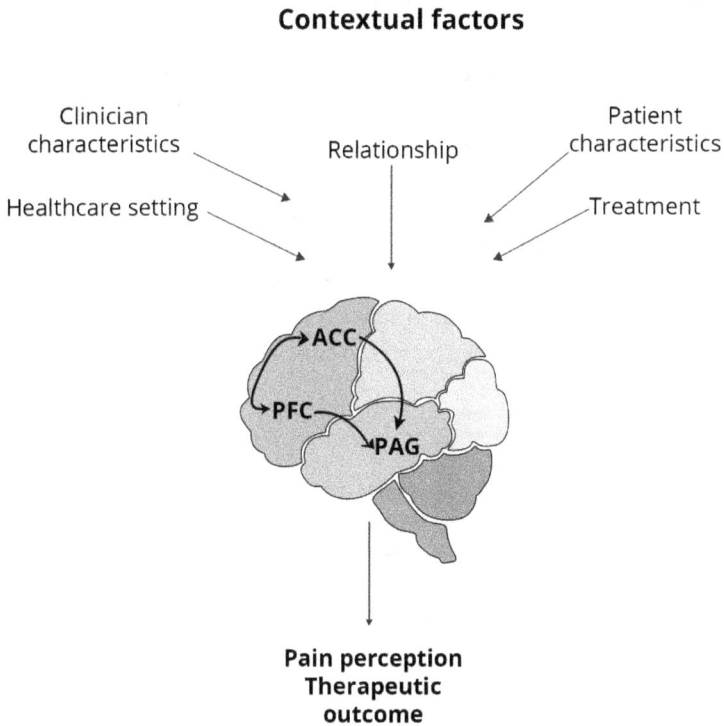

**Figure 7. Psycho-neurobiological mechanism of contextual factors.** Abbreviation: ACC = Anterior Cingulate Cortex; PFC = Prefrontal Cortex; PAG = Periaqueductal. Adapted under the terms of the Creative Commons Attribution 4.0 International License from Rossettini G, Carlino E, Testa M. Clinical relevance of contextual factors as triggers of placebo and nocebo effects in musculoskeletal pain. BMC Musculoskelet Disord.(5)

The impact of contextual factors on outcomes in MSK disorders is reported for a wide range of MSK conditions, such as low back pain, neck pain, shoulder pain, osteoarthritis, rheumatoid arthritis, and fibromyalgia.(5) The impact of contextual factors was measured for different MSK conditions and treatments. In fibromyalgia, 45% of the active drug treatment is attributed to contextual effect.(9) Relevant contextual effects of drug therapy in the treatment of non-specific low back pain have been reported.(10) In osteoarthritis, 75% of the overall treatment effect is attributable to contextual effects, rather than specific effects of treatments.(7),(11) In low back pain, 81% of the change in pain variance in acute pain, and 66% in chronic pain, following spinal manual therapies, can be ascribed to contextual effects.(12)

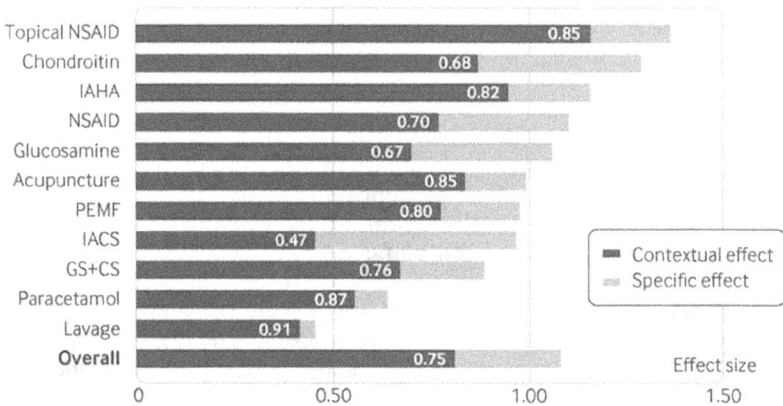

**Figure 8. Overall treatment effect and proportion attributable to contextual effect for pain in osteoarthritis.** CS = chondroitin sulfate; GS = glucosamine sulfate; IACS = intra-articular corticosteroid; IAHA = intra-articular hyaluronic acid; NSAID = non-steroidal anti-inflammatory drug; PEMF = pulsed electromagnetic field therapy. Reprinted with permission from author from Kaptchuk TJ, Hemond CC, Miller FG. Placebos in chronic pain: evidence, theory, ethics, and use in clinical practice. BMJ. 2020;370:m1668. doi:10.1136/bmj.m1668.(7)

Expectations and conditioning are important factors in the modulation of contextual effects on pain perception and treatment outcomes. The neurophysiologic mechanisms involved in this modulation can be explained with the predictive processing model (see chapter: Predictive Processing). A patient receiving an acute bottom-up nociceptive signal, with no previous exposure to the painful stimulus, will not have any top-down nociceptive predictions about the pain. Therefore, the pain perception will match the nociceptive input.(7)

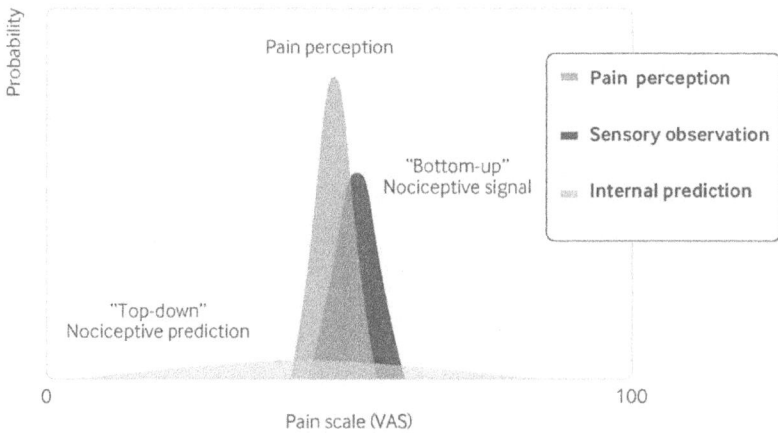

**Figure 9. Healthy normal predictive processing model of acute pain perception.** This is characterized by a lack of prior pain prediction (orange), yielding congruence between the sensory signal (blue) and perception (green). VAS = visual analog scale. Adapted with permission from author from Kaptchuk TJ, Hemond CC, Miller FG. Placebos in chronic pain: evidence, theory, ethics, and use in clinical practice. BMJ. 2020;370:m1668. doi:10.1136/bmj.m1668.(7)

A patient undergoing the same acute painful experience, but given a verbal suggestion that the pain will be of low intensity, will have an expectation about the nociceptive stimulus. This expectation leads to a top-down nociceptive prediction that will modulate the pain perception toward less pain.

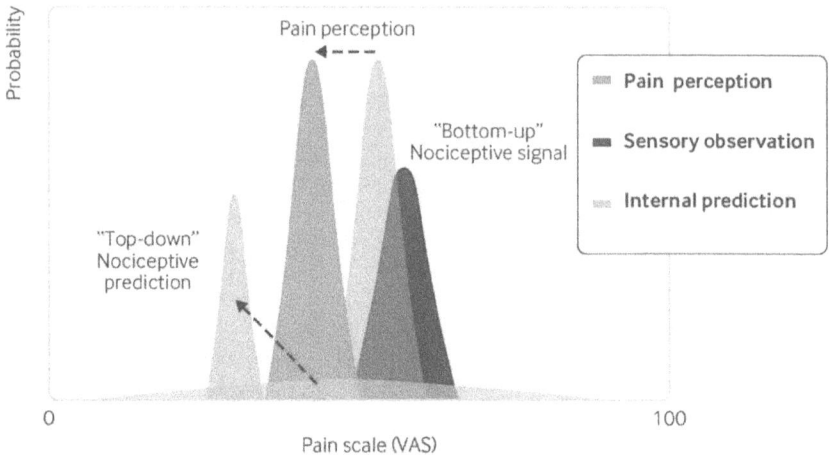

**Figure 10. Placebo hypoalgesia of acute experimental pain** can be modulated in healthy people via a temporary expectation-prediction lower in intensity than the painful stimulus. VAS = visual analog scale. Adapted with permission from author from Kaptchuk TJ, Hemond CC, Miller FG. Placebos in chronic pain: evidence, theory, ethics, and use in clinical practice. BMJ. 2020;370:m1668. doi:10.1136/bmj.m1668.(7)

Chronic pain can change the structural and functional architecture of the sensory and central processing pathways in such a way, that high-level top-down predictions shift incoming lower-level sensory data toward painful perception.(7) Therefore, lower intensity bottom-up nociceptive signals are perceived as more painful.

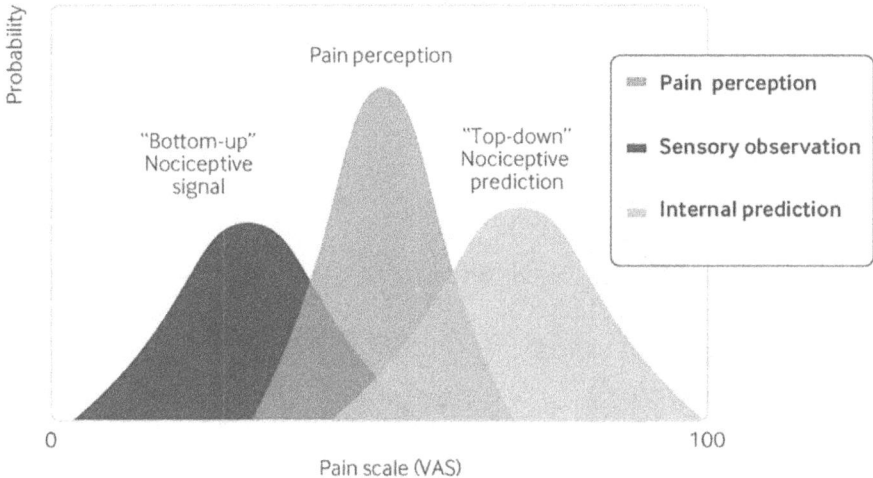

**Figure 11. Predictive processing model of chronic pain perception.** Account of chronic pain is characterized by upregulated prior (orange) prediction of incoming sensory (blue) signals. The predictive processing summation of these two signals yields a perception in between the two. VAS = visual analog scale. Adapted with permission from author from Kaptchuk TJ, Hemond CC, Miller FG. Placebos in chronic pain: evidence, theory, ethics, and use in clinical practice. BMJ. 2020;370:m1668. doi:10.1136/bmj.m1668.(7)

Contextual factors, such as a positive expectation for a novel therapeutic intervention, or reassurance from an empathic physician, can decrease these biased high-level top-down predictions and lead to decreased pain perception.(7) Contextual factors modulating effects on pain perception and treatment outcomes are mediated by high-level top-down processes.(7)

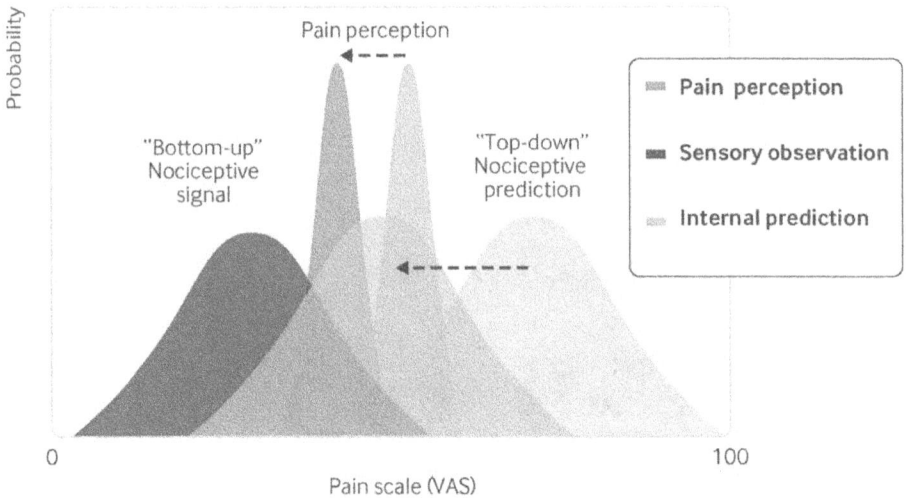

**Figure 12. Placebo effect in chronic pain.** Hypoalgesia can be achieved by shifting top-down predictions to more benign intensities. VAS = visual analog scale. Adapted with permission from author from Kaptchuk TJ, Hemond CC, Miller FG. Placebos in chronic pain: evidence, theory, ethics, and use in clinical practice. BMJ. 2020;370:m1668. doi:10.1136/bmj.m1668.(7)

Contextual factors play an important role in a patient's symptoms and outcomes. Contextual factors are linked to a lot of the same biophysiological mechanisms involved in patient and clinician dispositions, which shows the extensive interconnectivity of all the domains involved in the clinical encounter and management outcomes in MSK disorders.

Clinicians involved in the management of MSK disorders, need to understand contextual factors in order to use positive contexts, and avoid negative contexts, to potentialize the effectiveness of management strategies.

The social interactions, the therapeutic ritual, and the awareness of the ongoing procedure, are essential elements to take into consideration.(5) A pleasant and peaceful waiting room, with friendly and helpful staff, can help patients feel comfortable.(5) The therapeutic setting also plays an important role in maximizing contextual effects of therapy. The healthcare environment (e.g. light, color, design of the room) should make patients feel secure and comfortable. The social interaction between patients should focus on the positive effects of therapy, not the experience of negative outcomes (see Appendix B).(5)

Clinicians should assess a patient's previous experience, expectations, and beliefs by giving the patient the opportunity and the time to tell their story (see chapter: Communication). Clinicians should thoroughly examine their patients, and provide explanations of their conditions and treatment options that can be easily understood by patients. Patients should be motivated to be involved in the choice of therapy and treatment goals.(5) In such cases, patients will feel valued and understood, which will foster a positive, patient-centered, therapeutic alliance, a better patient-clinician relationship, and improved therapeutic outcomes. History-taking and a physical exam are associated with therapeutic effects related to pain, fear-avoidance, pain catastrophizing, and functional measures of mobility and sensitivity.(13)

# References

1. Carlino E, Benedetti F. Different contexts, different pains, different experiences. *Neuroscience*. 2016;338:19–26. doi:10.1016/j.neuroscience.2016.01.053

2. Bingel U. Placebo 2.0: the impact of expectations on analgesic treatment outcome. *Pain*. 2020;161 Suppl 1:S48–S56. doi:10.1097/j.pain.0000000000001981

3. Benedetti F. Placebo and the new physiology of the doctor-patient relationship. *Physiol Rev*. 2013;93(3):1207-1246. doi:10.1152/physrev.00043.2012

4. Perfitt JS, Plunkett N, Jones S. Placebo effect in the management of chronic pain. *BJA Educ*. 2020;20(11):382-387. doi:10.1016/j.bjae.2020.07.002

5. Rossettini G, Carlino E, Testa M. Clinical relevance of contextual factors as triggers of placebo and nocebo effects in musculoskeletal pain. *BMC Musculoskelet Disord*. 2018;19:27. doi:10.1186/s12891-018-1943-8

6. Zunhammer M, Spisák T, Wager TD, et al; Placebo Imaging Consortium. Meta-analysis of neural systems underlying placebo analgesia from individual participant fMRI data. *Nat Commun*. 2021;12:1391. doi:10.1038/s41467-021-21179-3

7. Kaptchuk TJ, Hemond CC, Miller FG. Placebos in chronic pain: evidence, theory, ethics, and use in clinical practice. *BMJ*. 2020;370:m1668. doi:10.1136/bmj.m1668

8. Sawicki CM, Humeidan ML, Sheridan JF. Neuroimmune interactions in pain and stress: an interdisciplinary approach. *Neuroscientist*. 2021;27(2):113-128. doi:10.1177/1073858420914747

9. Häuser W, Bartram-Wunn E, Bartram C, et al. Systematic review: placebo response in drug trials of fibromyalgia syndrome and painful peripheral diabetic neuropathy-magnitude and patient-related predictors. *Pain*. 2011;152(8):1709-1717. doi:10.1016/j.pain.2011.01.050

10. Puhl AA, Reinhart CJ, Rok ER, et al. An examination of the observed placebo effect associated with the treatment of low back pain - a systematic review. *Pain Res Manag*. 2011;16:45-52. doi:10.1155/2011/625315

11. Zou K, Wong J, Abdullah N, et al. Examination of overall treatment effect and the proportion attributable to contextual effect in osteoarthritis: meta-analysis of randomised controlled trials. *Ann Rheum Dis*. 2016;75(11):1964-1970. doi:10.1136/annrheumdis-2015-208387

12. Menke JM. Do manual therapies help low back pain? A comparative effectiveness meta-analysis. *Spine*. 2014;39(7):e463-e472. doi:10.1097/BRS.0000000000000230

13. Darlow B, Dean S, Perry M, et al. Easy to harm, hard to heal: patient views about the back. *Spine*. 2015;40(11):842-850. doi:10.1097/BRS.0000000000000901

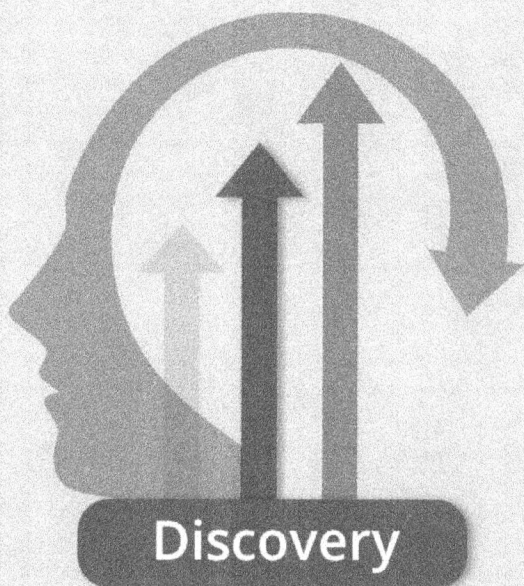
Discovery

# The Patient

# The Self

—⚭—

Chronic pain not only changes the structural and functional architecture of the sensory and central processing pathway of pain modulation,(1) but also changes a patient's conceptualization of themselves and their environment. (2) Individuals construct mental representations of the situations in which they find themselves (the context), in order to make sense of what they are experiencing. These conceptual representation models (self-in-context models) allow people to assign personal meaning to events and integrate them into current and future well-being.(2) Conceptual representations play an essential role in the predictive and regulatory functions of the brain, and therefore drive behavior and physiological responses in the body, affecting mental and physical health.(2) Self-in-context models infer the current physical and mental state, and predict behaviors and physiological regulations in response to internal (interoceptive) and external (exteroceptive) inputs based on predictive codes.(2) The representation models and the predictive codes are continuously updated by learning from prediction errors and are, therefore, influenced by contextual factors (see chapter: Predictive Processing).

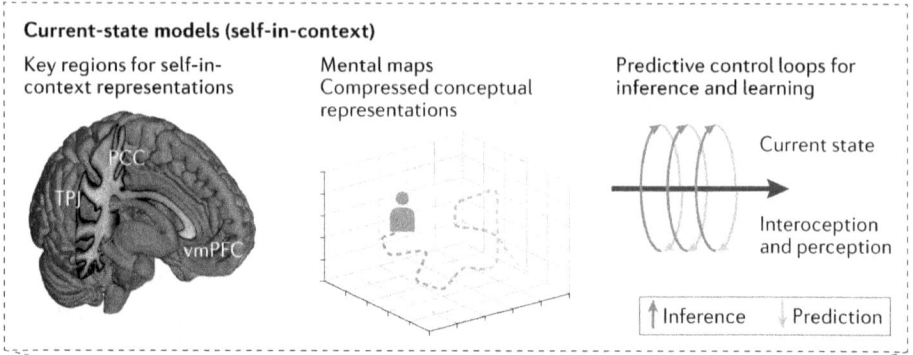

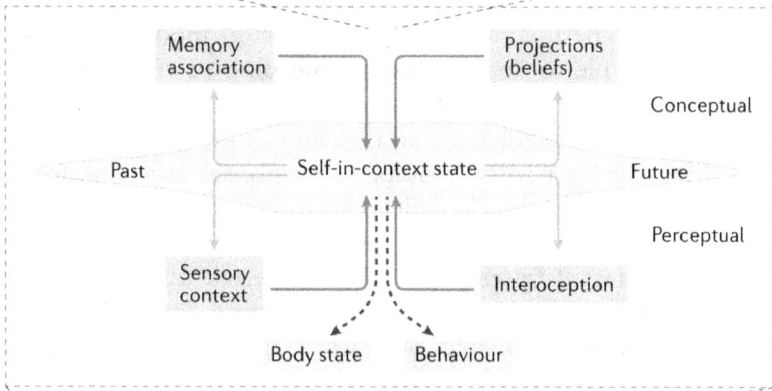

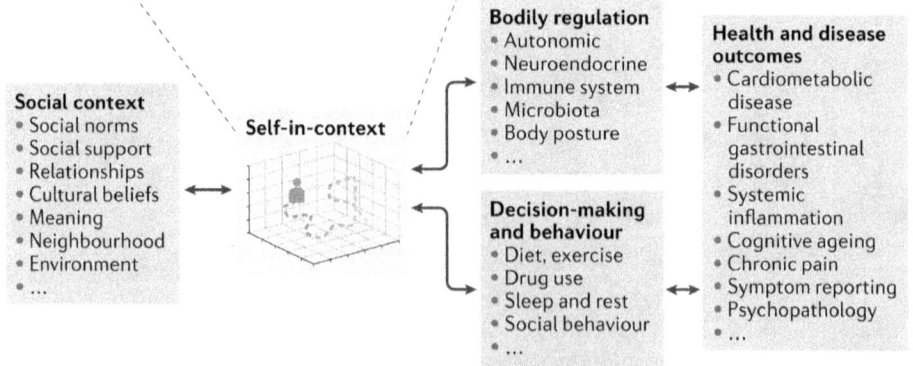

**Figure 13. A schematic of self-in-context models and their role in health and disease.** The ventromedial prefrontal cortex (vmPFC), together with other key regions of the default-mode network, such as the temporoparietal junction (TPJ) and posterior cingulate cortex (PCC), locates the current position of the self in a compressed low-dimensional space that captures the essential features of a situation. Locating the current state of the self on a mental or conceptual map is central to the process of "meaning-making". "Self-in-context" models are inference-based models of the current state that predict sensory and interoceptive input and guide behavior and physiological regulation on the basis of predictive codes. They also shape and are shaped by beliefs, associative memory and learning. Self-in-context models are influenced by the social and environmental context of the agent, including but not limited to social norms, relationships, cultural beliefs and neighbourhood characteristics. In turn, they can regulate visceral outflow via vmPFC projections to the hypothalamus and the brainstem. Self-in-context models also influence decision-making and health-relevant behavior (for example, dietary choices and how one works and connects with others) via vmPFC connections with the basal ganglia and the mesolimbic reward circuit or frontostriatal loops. Together, the dual pathways — influences on bodily physiology and decision-making — can exert long-term effects on mental and bodily health in multiple ways, such as via their effects on inflammation and allostasis, or their interactions with other health-relevant systems, such as microbiota (for example, via dietary patterns). For instance, maladaptive thought patterns and self-in-context models may lead to a dysregulation of the autonomic nervous system, which leads to allostatic load and diminished recovery, with long-term effects on bodily organs. At the same time, self-in-context models may lead to changes in health-related behavior such as unhealthy food choices, drug use or insufficient exercise, which also impact health in the short term and the long term. Reprinted with permission from publisher from Koban L, Gianaros PJ, Kober H, et al. The self in context: brain systems linking mental and physical health. Nat Rev Neurosci.

The generation of conceptual mental models of self, requires the connection of multiple, large-scale, brain networks (default-mode network, salience network, limbic network, and frontoparietal network) in which the default-mode network, and in particular, the prefrontal cortex, plays a vital role. (2),(3) The ventromedial prefrontal cortex is at the center of the structural and functional interaction of connected brain networks.

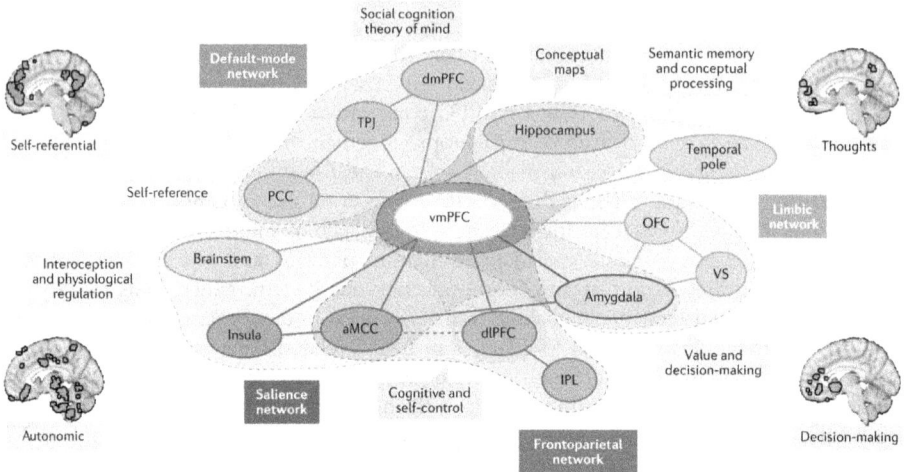

**Figure 14. Functional associations of ventromedial prefrontal cortex with connected brain networks.** The ventromedial prefrontal cortex (vmPFC) is closely connected to areas of the default-mode network. Together with other regions of the default-mode network, including the temporoparietal junction (TPJ), the dorsomedial prefrontal cortex (dmPFC), the hippocampus and the posterior cingulate cortex (PCC), it is involved in social cognition and self-referential thought. Both the hippocampus and the vmPFC show evidence for grid-like coding of spatial and conceptual maps, and together with other temporal and frontal areas are involved in semantic memory and conceptual processing more broadly. The most ventral part of the vmPFC is connected to the limbic network, including the orbitofrontal cortex (OFC), the ventral striatum (VS), and other subcortical areas. Together with the VS, the vmPFC is important for reward processing and decision-making. Therefore, it is amenable to interactions with the frontoparietal network, especially the dorsolateral prefrontal cortex (dlPFC) and the inferior parietal lobule (IPL), involved in executive function and self-control. Together with areas of the salience network (especially the anterior midcingulate cortex (aMCC) and the anterior insula) and subcortical regions, the vmPFC is involved in interoception and physiological regulation. Representative Neurosynth term-based-meta-analytic association maps (with a threshold at false discovery rate q < 0.01, reproducible and available for download from https://neurosynth.org) illustrate the role of the vmPFC with self-referential processing, conceptual thoughts, decision-making and autonomic regulation. Reprinted with permission from publisher from Koban L, Gianaros PJ, Kober H, et al. The self in context: brain systems linking mental and physical health. Nat Rev Neurosci.

Therefore, the ventromedial prefrontal cortex, through its structural and functional associations with connected brain networks, has far-reaching implications for mental and physical well-being (see Appendix C).

The prefrontal cortex also influences descending pain modulation (see chapter: Contextual Dispositions); psychological behaviors, such as depression (see chapter: Depression) and reward mechanisms (see chapter: Pain Catastrophizing); immunity, including inflammation (see chapter: Metabolic Health); and autonomic and neuroendocrine responses (see chapter: Metabolic Health).(2) The prefrontal cortex also encodes attitudes related to racial stereotypes, and is related to higher pain sensitivity in African-Americans (see chapter: Culture).(2)

The alterations in self-in-context representations and sense-making processes in chronic pain, are associated with structural and functional alterations in the ventromedial prefrontal cortex and the default-mode network, underlining their neurophysiological connectedness.(2) Maladaptive self-in-context models will influence pain perception and behavior, in patients suffering from MSK disorders. Conversely, self-in-context models are shaped by contextual dispositions whose mechanisms are key in understanding patient experience. On the other hand, the adaptive nature of the conceptual representation models and predictive codes allow for therapeutic interventions, such as activities that promote purpose, self-efficacy, feelings of connection to others, social engagement, meditation, mindful acceptance, and positive treatment expectancies.(2)

## References

1. Kaptchuk TJ, Hemond CC, Miller FG. Placebos in chronic pain: evidence, theory, ethics, and use in clinical practice. *BMJ*. 2020;370:m1668. doi:10.1136/bmj.m1668

2. Koban L, Gianaros PJ, Kober H, et al. The self in context: brain systems linking mental and physical health. *Nat Rev Neurosci*. 2021;22:309–322. doi:10.1038/s41583-021-00446-8

3. Geuter S, Koban L, Wager TD. The cognitive neuroscience of placebo effects: concepts, predictions, and physiology. *Annu Rev Neurosci*. 2017;40:167-188. doi:10.1146/annurev-neuro-072116-031132

# Culture

Cultural factors influence the quality of health services provided to patients. Minority populations have a different set of attitudes, beliefs, and expectations that, if unrecognized and unmet, can lead to poor health care delivery. Therefore, clinicians need to take cultural factors into consideration during the clinical encounter with patients affected by MSK disorders.

Culture incorporates layers of ethnicity, race, nationality, religion, regionalism, family, and group memberships (e.g. work or hobby groups).(1) Each layer of culture influences a patient's view of health and medicine.(1)

Communication is affected by cultural disposition. Miscommunication happens not only through words and phrases, but also at the deeper level of values and beliefs.(1) Language differences between clinicians, patients, and their families, affect the health literacy of patients and their family in understanding their disorder, communication with clinicians, and navigating the health care system.(1) Language barriers, lack of access to interpreting services, cultural differences in communication style, and health literacy, impact patient-clinician communication, treatment adherence, and outcomes. (2)

The burden of pain is unequal across cultural groups.(3) The experience of pain, and the assessment and treatment of pain, are influenced by racial and ethnic differences.(2),(4) The difference in the experience of pain may be driven by differences in pain coping methods, especially when it comes to catastrophizing, praying, or stoicism.(2),(4) Perceived bias and discrimination can lead to increased experimental and clinical pain among minorities.(2) Racial and ethnic minority patients have worse pain expectations which can influence pain perception and treatment outcomes.(2) Pain-related disability is higher in patients from minority groups.(5),(6) Ethnic minorities bear a disproportionate burden of pain that, in part, originates from differences in the internal valuation of pain.(7) Different populations with chronic MSK disorders exhibit different coping strategies, illness perceptions, self-efficacy, fear-avoidance beliefs, locus of control, and pain attitudes.(8)

Cultural differences among people of diverse backgrounds lead to different pain treatment preferences.(2) Patients from different cultural backgrounds might prefer prescription medication treatment for pain, while others will rather seek chiropractic care, physical therapy, creams and ointments, electric blankets, folk remedies, or yoga.(2) Preferences in surgery for the management of osteoarthritis can also differ from one culture to the other. Patients from specific cultural backgrounds perceive alternative treatment, such as prayer, and are less willing to undergo total knee arthroplasty.(2) The utilization of pain medicine might be perceived as a sign of weakness within certain communities, where remaining stoic serves to save face.(2) Fear of addiction and side-effects from pain medication is bigger in some cultures and can also influence treatment preference.(2)

Neurophysiological mechanisms also differ between cultural groups and explain, in part, differences in pain perception. Some minority groups have reduced nociceptive flexion reflex thresholds, increased temporal summation of heat pain, reduced conditioned pain modulation, and reduced diffuse noxious inhibitory controls contributing to ethnic disparities in experimental and clinical pain.(9) Other endogenous pain regulatory mechanisms differ between ethnic groups as well. The levels and function of hormones and neurotransmitters, such as norepinephrine, cortisol, oxytocin, endorphins, and allopregnanolone have been shown to differ in different ethnic groups. (9) Some of these endogenous pain regulatory mechanisms function less efficiently in some ethnic groups, therefore impacting pain perception in those groups.(9) Higher levels of reported pain amongst minority groups may also arise from differences in extra-nociceptive brain systems implicated in modulation, valuation, and chronification of pain.(7)

Clinicians need to be aware of and understand the cultural mechanisms involved in the pain presentation of patients from minority groups. Strategies to mitigate discrepancies in the assessment and treatment of MSK disorders in minority populations need to be implemented. Clinicians need to become culturally competent in their delivery of care.

# References

1. O'Toole JK, Alvarado-Little W, Ledford CJ. Communication with diverse patients: addressing culture and language. *Pediatr Clin North Am*. 2019;66(4):791-804. doi:10.1016/j.pcl.2019.03.006

2. Meints SM, Cortes A, Morais CA, et al. Racial and ethnic differences in the experience and treatment of noncancer pain. *Pain Manag*. 2019;9(3):317-334. doi:10.2217/pmt-2018-0030

3. Brady B, Veljanova I, Chipchase L. The intersections of chronic noncancer pain: culturally diverse perspectives on disease burden. [Published correction appears in Pain Med. Oct 1, 2019;20(10):2080]. *Pain Med*. 2019;20(3):434-445. doi:10.1093/pm/pny088

4. Krupić F, Čustović S, Jašarević M, et al. Ethnic differences in the perception of pain: a systematic review of qualitative and quantitative research. *Med Glas (Zenica)*. 2019;16:108-114. doi:10.17392/966-19

5. Janevic MR, McLaughlin SJ, Heapy AA, et al. Racial and socioeconomic Ddsparities in disabling chronic pain: findings from the health and retirement study. *J Pain*. 2017;18(12):1459-1467. doi:10.1016/j.jpain.2017.07.005

6. Vaughn IA, Terry EL, Bartley EJ, et al. Racial-ethnic differences in osteoarthritis pain and disability: a meta-analysis. *J Pain*. 2019;20(6):629-644. doi:10.1016/j.jpain.2018.11.012

7. Losin EAR, Woo CW, Medina NA, et al. Neural and sociocultural mediators of ethnic differences in pain. [Published correction appears in Nat Hum Behav. Mar 3, 2020]. *Nat Hum Behav*. 2020;4(5):517-530. doi:10.1038/s41562-020-0819-8

8. Orhan C, Van Looveren E, Cagnie B, et al. Are pain beliefs, cognitions, and behaviors influenced by race, ethnicity, and culture in patients with chronic musculoskeletal pain: a systematic review. *Pain Physician*. 2018;21(6):541-558.

9. Campbell CM, Edwards RR. Ethnic differences in pain and pain management. *Pain Manag*. 2012;2(3):219-230. doi:10.2217/pmt.12.7

# Social Determinants of Health

Social determinants define the conditions in which people are born, grow, live, work, and age, and the inequities in power, money, and resources involved in disparities in health outcomes. Social determinants play an important role in MSK care and are often overlooked by MSK clinicians.

The risk of chronic pain is increased with low and medium socioeconomic status compared with high socioeconomic status.(1) An Odds Ratio of 1.32 and 1.16 respectively were found for low and medium socioeconomic status, as compared with high level status.(1)

Educational attainment, insurance type, and employment status are strong predictors of clinical outcomes in patients undergoing primary lumbar surgery.(2)

Education status, socioeconomic status (low income, unemployment), and occupational factors (manual lifting, working overtime, lack of supporting staff, and low job satisfaction), are associated with worse outcomes in chronic low back pain (LBP).(3),(4) Chronic pain patients in the lowest wealth quartile report more pain-related disability.(5) Educational attainment and socioeconomic status show the strongest relationship between social determinants of health and chronic LBP.(3)

Limited access to education, access to poor quality education, limited language proficiency, learning differences and disabilities, and cognitive impairment lead to limited health literacy. Patients with limited health literacy are more likely to have poor health, higher rates of chronic disease, and a mortality rate nearly double that of a patient who has adequate health literacy. Persons with limited health literacy are more likely to experience disparities in health care access and show worse adherence and inadequate skills for managing their disorder.(6)

Early life experience and stress affect nociception, mood, and pain behaviors throughout life.(7) Violence, including adverse childhood experiences, intimate partner violence, and elder abuse, also have an impact on health disparities.(8) Persons who report abusive or neglectful childhood experiences are at increased risk of experiencing chronic pain later in life.(9),(10),(11) Abuse history is also linked to poorer self-reported health and greater negative affect.(11) Childhood abuse and neglect are strongly associated with depression and anxiety.(12)

Between 5% and 30% of emerging adults (aged 18 to 29 years) suffer from chronic pain.(13) Familial chronic pain, previous chronic pain in childhood, history of abuse, sleep problems, anxiety and depression, and stress are factors associated with chronic pain in emerging adults.(13) Consequences from chronic pain in emerging adults can be devastating and include interruption to study and work, poorer physical functioning, and pain-related interference to socializing.(13) The management of emerging adults is rendered complicated by the perception of the health care system that is seen as outdated, and by competing priorities among pain treatment, educational requirements, and occupational commitments.(13) Management of emerging adults should take into account age-relevant topics, such as sexual health and the role of sleep in pain.(13)

Physically demanding work increases the risk of developing MSK disorders during working life. Job demands in early working life, such as standing or walking with lifting and carrying, and heavy or fast physically strenuous work, increase the likelihood of poor MSK health later in working life.(14) Chronic LBP, for instance, is related to increased workload, low job control, and poor social support.(15)

Pain is one of the most commonly reported symptoms in the aging population, but is often undertreated.(16) Pain does not constitute part of the normal aging process, contrary to beliefs among patients and physicians. (16),(17) The management of pain in the older population is rendered difficult by issues assessing pain in geriatric patients, the complexities of multiple comorbidities, and the high prevalence of polypharmacy.(16),(17) Older people do show unique characteristics of pain, including decreased pain to acute pathologies, increased pain threshold, decreased pain tolerance, prolonged and impaired recovery from tissue and nerve injury, and age-specific inter-relationships of psychosocial factors important in the adjustment to chronic pain. (17),(18) Neurophysiological response to tissue injury changes with age and is associated with prolonged inflammation and impaired recovery.(18) Changes in neuropathophysiology, neuroimmunological response, and the integrity of endogenous pain inhibitory systems affect geriatric pain.(18) A systemic pro-inflammatory state (inflammageing) is typical of aging itself and is associated with adipose tissue changes.(19) Aging is associated with core geriatric syndromes, including frailty, functional decline, susceptibility to increased disability, and symptom burdens that all play a role in MSK pain. (18) The elderly are more likely to suffer from both pain and depression, whereas pain severity is strongly associated with depression in that population. (20) Pain assessment in older adults needs to consider the unique features of the geriatric patient and the clinical encounter must be tailored to the needs of that population. Asking people about their pain is considered the most accurate and reliable assessment,(21) but is complicated in the geriatric population as older patients can have difficulties understanding the request, recalling the pain, or interpreting the painful signal.(21) The observation of specific pain behaviors is advocated when communication and cognitive function are impaired.(21) Pain assessment tools are available to facilitate the clinical encounter in the aging population.(21)

A social network is an important component of the determination of overall health and is associated with outcomes in MSK disorders. The impact of the social network on pain depends on the connectedness and the quality of interpersonal interactions.(22) Social presence alone is not associated with a reduction in pain intensity and pain sensitivity.(23) The presence of a significant other, increases facial expression of pain and increases physiological response to pain.(23) The presence of a stranger does not influence pain perception or expression.(23) These findings suggest that increased pain expression and response, serve as triggers for empathy and social support from significant others, and bears evolutionary importance. (23) Pain reduction relies not only on physical presence but, more importantly, on the perceived support from the companion.(22),(23) Communication becomes central to the perceived support and pain reduction. Indeed, verbal support decreases pain experience and physiological responses to pain. (23) The analgesic effect of verbal support requires positive and structured communication.(23) The modulating effect of verbal support on pain, relies on the increase in intimacy and/or emotion regulation which results in a decrease in perceived threat and stress.(22),(23) This effect is modulated by oxytocin, a neuropeptide that promotes intimacy and social interactions.(23) The importance of intimacy and connectedness is further demonstrated by social touch. Social touch by a romantic partner has an evident analgesic effect, whereas social touch by a stranger does not.(23) Social touch from a significant other, attenuates body arousal and threat-related brain activation, and promotes communication of emotions leading to stress control and pain reduction.(23) Pain reduction achieved through social support also promotes participation in physical activity by people suffering from pain. (24) A higher level of moderate-intensity physical activity is associated with better overall health and decreased pain (see chapter: Physical Activity). Support from significant others in the form of verbal interactions including encouragement, emotional validation, and reinterpretation, as well as from physical interactions (e.g. touch, mutual activities) provide support therapies for the management of pain.(22),(23) A patient's evaluation of their social networks needs to focus not solely on the quantity but, more significantly, on the quality of their network.

MSK clinicians need to ask their patients about social determinants of health in order to get a full picture of the patient's situation, and to discuss and address these dispositions and their influence on their disorder. Proposed topics for taking a more complete social history are described in Appendix D: Social History.(8)

# References

1. Prego-Domínguez J, Khazaeipour Z, Mallah N, et al. Socioeconomic status and occurrence of chronic pain: a meta-analysis. *Rheumatology (Oxford)*. 2021;60(3):1091-1105. doi:10.1093/rheumatology/keaa758

2. Rethorn ZD, Garcia AN, Cook CE, et al. Quantifying the collective influence of social determinants of health using conditional and cluster modeling. *PLoS One*. 2020;15(11):e0241868. doi:10.1371/journal.pone.0241868

3. Karran EL, Grant AR, Moseley GL. Low back pain and the social determinants of health: a systematic review and narrative synthesis. *Pain*. 2020;161(11):2476-2493. doi:10.1097/j.pain.0000000000001944

4. Wami SD, Abere G, Dessie A, et al. Work-related risk factors and the prevalence of low back pain among low wage workers: results from a cross-sectional study. *BMC Public Health*. 2019;19:1072. doi:10.1186/s12889-019-7430-9

5. Janevic MR, McLaughlin SJ, Heapy AA, et al. Racial and socioeconomic disparities in disabling chronic pain: findings from the health and retirement study. *J Pain*. 2017;18(12):1459-1467. doi:10.1016/j.jpain.2017.07.005

6. Schillinger D. The intersections between social determinants of health, health literacy, and health disparities. *Stud Health Technol Inform*. 2020;269:22-41. doi:10.3233/shti200020

7. Karshikoff B, Tadros MA, Mackey S, et al. Neuroimmune modulation of pain across the developmental spectrum. *Curr Opin Behav Sci*. 2019;28:85-92. doi:10.1016/j.cobeha.2019.01.010

8. Andermann A. Screening for social determinants of health in clinical care: moving from the margins to the mainstream. *Public Health Rev.* 2018;39:19. doi:10.1186/s40985-018-0094-7

9. Davis DA, Luecken LJ, Zautra AJ. Are reports of childhood abuse related to the experience of chronic pain in adulthood? A meta-analytic review of the literature. *Clin J Pain.* 2005;21(5):398-405. doi:10.1097/01.ajp.0000149795.08746.31

10. Brown J, Berenson K, Cohen P. Documented and self-reported child abuse and adult pain in a community sample. *Clin J Pain.* 2005;21(5):374-377. doi:10.1097/01.ajp.0000149797.16370.dc

11. Fillingim RB, Edwards RR. Is self-reported childhood abuse history associated with pain perception among healthy young women and men? *Clin J Pain.* 2005;21(5):387-397. doi:10.1097/01.ajp.0000149801.46864.39

12. Tietjen GE, Brandes JL, Peterlin BL, et al. Childhood maltreatment and migraine (part I). Prevalence and adult revictimization: a multicenter headache clinic survey. *Headache.* 2010;50:20-31. doi:10.1111/j.1526-4610.2009.01556.x

13. Brown D, Schenk S, Genent D, et al. A scoping review of chronic pain in emerging adults. *PAIN Reports.* 6:e920. doi:10.1097/pr9.0000000000000920

14. Bláfoss R, Skovlund SV, López-Bueno R, et al. Is hard physical work in the early working life associated with back pain later in life? A cross-sectional study among 5700 older workers. *BMJ Open.* 2020;10(12):e040158. doi:10.1136/bmjopen-2020-040158

15. Buruck G, Tomaschek A, Wendsche J, et al. Psychosocial areas of worklife and chronic low back pain: a systematic review and meta-analysis. *BMC Musculoskelet Disord.* 2019;20:480. doi:10.1186/s12891-019-2826-3

16. Borsheski R, Johnson QL. Pain management in the geriatric population. *Mo Med.* 2014;111(6):508-511.

17. Bicket MC, Mao J. Chronic pain in older adults. *Anesthesiol Clin.* 2015;33(3):577-590. doi:10.1016/j.anclin.2015.05.011

18. Gagliese L. Pain and aging: the emergence of a new subfield of pain research. *J Pain.* 2009;10(4):343-353. doi:10.1016/j.jpain.2008.10.013

19. Zamboni M, Nori N, Brunelli A, et al. How does adipose tissue contribute to inflammageing? *Exp Gerontol.* 2021;143:111-162. doi:10.1016/j.exger.2020.111162

20. Zis P, Daskalaki A, Bountouni I, et al. Depression and chronic pain in the elderly: links and management challenges. *Clin Interv Aging.* 2017;12:709-720. doi:10.2147/cia.S113576

21. Gregory J. The complexity of pain assessment in older people. *Nurs Older People.* 2015;27(8):16-21. doi:10.7748/nop.27.8.16.e738

22. Fernández-Peña R, Molina JL, Valero O. Satisfaction with social support received from social relationships in cases of chronic pain: the influence of personal network characteristics in terms of structure, composition and functional content. *Int J Environ Res Public Health*. 2020;17(8):2706. doi:10.3390/ijerph17082706

23. Che X, Cash R, Chung S, et al. Investigating the influence of social support on experimental pain and related physiological arousal: a systematic review and meta-analysis. *Neurosci Biobehav Rev*. 2018;92:437-452. doi:10.1016/j.neubiorev.2018.07.005

24. Stevens M, Cruwys T, Murray K. Social support facilitates physical activity by reducing pain. *Br J Health Psychol*. 2020;25(3):576-595. doi:10.1111/bjhp.12424

# Health Literacy

Health literacy is defined as the cognitive and social skills which determine the motivation and ability of individuals to gain access to, understand, and use information in ways that promote and maintain good health.(1) Health literacy is linked to the social determinants of health. Inadequate health literacy is associated with older age, lower socioeconomic status, lower education, mental health status, and increased comorbidities.(2)

Limited health literacy is linked to poor health outcomes.(3),(4) Limited health literacy disproportionally affects vulnerable populations, such as the elderly, the disabled, people of lower socioeconomic status, ethnic minorities, people with limited language proficiency, and people with limited education. (2),(3),(5)

People with limited health literacy are more likely to experience disparities in health care access, including less screening and preventative services, and are more likely to have poor health, higher rates of chronic disease, and nearly double the mortality rate.(3)

Health literacy is negatively associated with current opioid misuse, the severity of opioid dependency, pain severity, and pain disability.(6) Patients with MSK disorders who have inadequate health literacy, experience lower physical function and higher pain intensity.(2),(7) The differences in physical function and pain scores increase over time in patients with inadequate health literacy.(2) Patients with poorer self-efficacy, benefit less from self-management of MSK disorders, as such management strategies require a high level of patient participation and engagement.(2),(4) Patients with lower levels of health literacy show greater catastrophizing and lower pain-related self-efficacy.(5),(8)

Patients with limited health literacy exhibit worse management adherence and inadequate skills for managing their disorders.(2),(3),(4) Limited health literacy also has a negative effect on clinician-patient communication.(3) Patients with limited health literacy use a more passive communication style, are less likely to engage in shared decision-making, and are more likely to report that interactions with their clinician are not helpful or empowering. (3) Furthermore, clinicians find pain management in patients with low health literacy challenging.(2)

Shared decision-making and patient empowerment are central elements of evidence-based management of MSK disorders. Therefore, clinicians involved in the management of MSK disorders must consider their patients' levels of health literacy. Communication and educational interventions must be adapted to the levels of understanding and knowledge of the patients.

In the context of patient-clinician communication, clinicians can implement a number of oral communication strategies informed by health literacy. The teach-back method is one of the most important universal precautions for health literacy.(9) The teach-back method consists of having the patient describe the information they have been given, using their own words. If the patient states ("teaches back") the information inaccurately or repeats the clinician's information word-for-word, the clinician re-teaches the information in a different way, then again asks for a teach-back of the information.(9) This is repeated until the patient can teach the information in his or her own words.(9) Teach-back can increase comprehension, reduce medication errors, and reduce hospital re-admissions.(9) A show-back method can be implemented for instructions about equipment use or performance of a technical skill.(9)

Another health-literacy-informed strategy clinicians can use for verbal communication, is to limit the amount of information presented at one time. (9) Verbal communication should be limited to two or three of the most important messages, reflecting the "need-to-know" information.(9) In the event of large quantities of "need-to-know" messages, teaching should be provided in several sittings, prioritizing the most important messages first.(9) Other strategies include speaking distinctly, speaking at a moderate pace, and using common, everyday language, free of medical jargon.(9)

Written information to supplement what is discussed verbally can help reduce cognitive load, making it easier for patients to understand and comply with the information provided.(9) Written material should incorporate plain language principles and include simple visual aids. The literature should make its purpose evident and concentrate on logically sequenced messages in limited numbers.(9)

# References

1. Britt RK, Collins WB, Wilson K, et al. eHealth literacy and health behaviors affecting modern college students: a pilot study of issues identified by the American College Health Association. *J Med Internet Res.* 2017;19(12):e392. doi:10.2196/jmir.3100

2. Lacey RJ, Campbell P, Lewis M, et al. The impact of inadequate health literacy in a population with musculoskeletal pain. *Health Lit Res Pract.* 2018;2(4):e215-e220. doi:10.3928/24748307-20181101-01

3. Schillinger D. The intersections between social determinants of health, health literacy, and health disparities. *Stud Health Technol Inform.* 2020;269:22-41. doi:10.3233/shtI200020

4. Edward J, Carreon LY, Williams MV, et al. The importance and impact of patients' health literacy on low back pain management: a systematic review of literature. *Spine J.* 2018;18(2):370-376. doi:10.1016/j.spinee.2017.09.005

5. Mackey LM, Blake C, Casey MB, et al. The impact of health literacy on health outcomes in individuals with chronic pain: a cross-sectional study. *Physiotherapy.* 2019;105(3):346-353. doi:10.1016/j.physio.2018.11.006

6. Rogers AH, Bakhshaie J, Orr MF, et al. Health literacy, opioid misuse, and pain experience among adults with chronic pain. *Pain Med.* 2020;21(4):670-676. doi:10.1093/pm/pnz062

7. Köppen PJ, Dorner TE, Stein KV, et al. Health literacy, pain intensity and pain perception in patients with chronic pain. *Wien Klin Wochenschr.* 2018;130:23–30. doi:10.1007/s00508-017-1309-5

8. Kapoor S, Eyer J, Thorn B. Health literacy in individuals with chronic pain living in rural United States: association with pain-related variables. *The Journal of Pain.* 2016;17:S17-S18. doi:10.1016/j.jpain.2016.01.071

9. Glick AF, Brach C, Yin HS, et al. Health literacy in the inpatient setting: implications for patient care and patient safety. *Pediatr Clin North Am.* 2019;66(4):805-826. doi:10.1016/j.pcl.2019.03.007

# Pain Catastrophizing

As described in The Common Sense Model chapter, the fear-avoidance model describes pain catastrophizing as a means of making sense of the pain experience.

Patients who catastrophize about symptoms associated with MSK disorders (including low back pain, knee osteoarthritis, hip osteoarthritis, Achilles tendinopathy, shoulder injury, peripheral MSK joint conditions) can embark on a set of negative cognitive, emotional, and behavioral responses. (1),(2),(3),(4),(5),(6),(7),(8) Pain catastrophizing, excessive fear response, and avoidance behaviors that are not proportional to the actual threat can be conditioned through direct experience by information (vicarious learning) or by observation (modeling).(9) Negative affect can also promote pain catastrophizing and pain control behavior, leading to more avoidance and disability.(10) Pain catastrophizing can lead to pain-related fear and activity avoidance, eventually resulting in disability (disuse and depression). Physical disability and depression, in turn, heightens the pain experience, and creates a vicious cycle.(9),(10),(11) On the other hand, the lack of catastrophizing and the confrontation of normal activity can lead to recovery.(9),(10),(11) Avoidance behavior, once acquired, is often persistent and difficult to overcome, and can be generalized to new situations that share features of the initial stimulus — leading to more pain-related fear, pain, and disability. (9),(10),(12),(13)

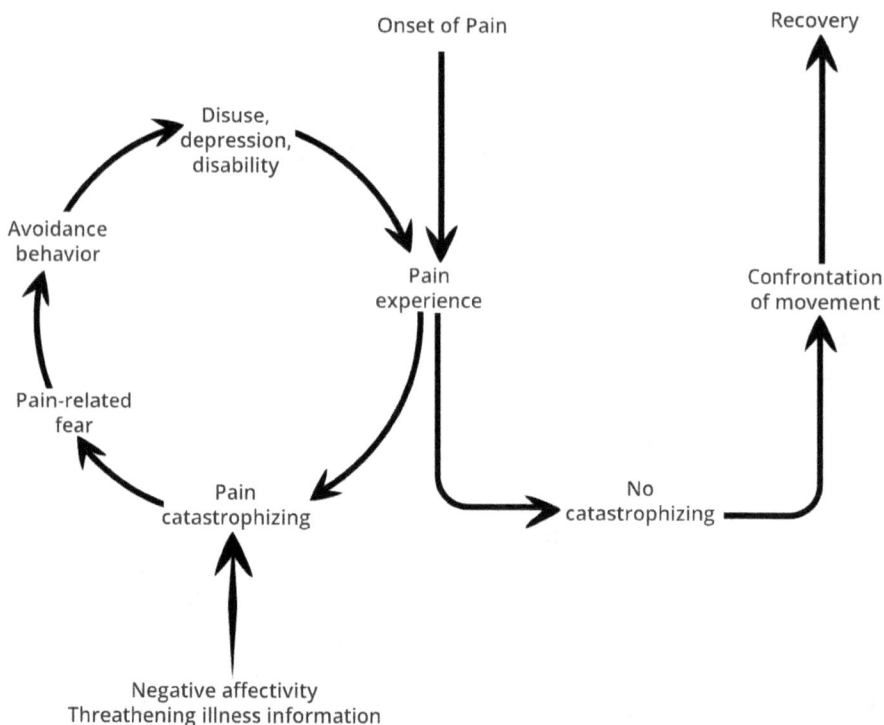

**Figure 15. Fear-avoidance model.** Reprinted with permission from publisher from Bunzli S, Smith A, Schütze R, et al. Making sense of low back pain and pain-related fear. J Orthop Sports Phys Ther. (11)

Pain catastrophizing is characterized by the magnification of the threat level of the painful stimulus, the helplessness felt in dealing with the pain experience, and the relative inability to suppress pain-related thoughts. (14) Pain catastrophizing is one of the most robust and reliable predictors of adverse pain experience.(14),(15) High levels of pain catastrophizing correlate with higher pain intensity, increased pain severity, and emotional distress.(14) Pain catastrophizing is a multifaceted complex construct that includes emotional regulation, catastrophic worry, neuropsychological models of personality traits, the behavioral inhibition system (BIS), and the behavioral activation system (BAS).(14)

Pain catastrophizing can be seen as repetitive, negative thinking, similar to worry, where the function is to decrease negative emotions triggered by pain and other related stimuli.(15) Therefore, worry is a central element of catastrophizing. Worry motivates patients to find solutions to their problem. When a solution does not work, more worry is generated to find new solutions.

Patients can find themselves trapped in a never-ending loop of misdirected problem-solving.(16) The never-ending loop of catastrophic worrying can lead to unhelpful cognitive and behavioral coping strategies that end up potentiating the problem instead of solving it. Patients find themselves stuck in a maladaptive passive-avoidant coping strategy (suppression of elicited emotions) instead of developing constructive concrete problem-solving (re-appraisal of elicited emotions).(14),(15),(17) Worry, as a persistent cognitive activity, deals with emotional material on a superficial, abstract level.(15) In the short run, worry can help to suppress aversive images and intense negative emotions, but in the long run, the cognitive avoidance of emotional processing leads to increased emotional problems (anxiety and depression) and disability.(15) Catastrophizing is, therefore, a form of an emotional regulatory process where cognitions, emotions, and behaviors are intertwined.

The next step in understanding the fear-avoidance model is to identify factors that make some individuals prone to undergoing catastrophic worry. Suppression (avoidance) and re-appraisal (approach) responses (emotions, cognitions, and behaviors) are rooted in two neurophysiological systems: the BIS and the BAS.(18),(19) Typically, acute pain activates the BAS by increasing dopamine transmission in the brain's reward and motivational centers. Chronic pain, on the other hand, stimulates the BIS and leads to diminished motivation and depression. Dysregulation in the processing of nociceptive information, such as catastrophic worry, from the periphery to higher cortical centers, can shift the pain response from BAS-dominant to BIS-dominant. The BIS-BAS model of pain is built in a hierarchical manner and is another example of predictive processing (see chapter: Predictive Processing) in pain.

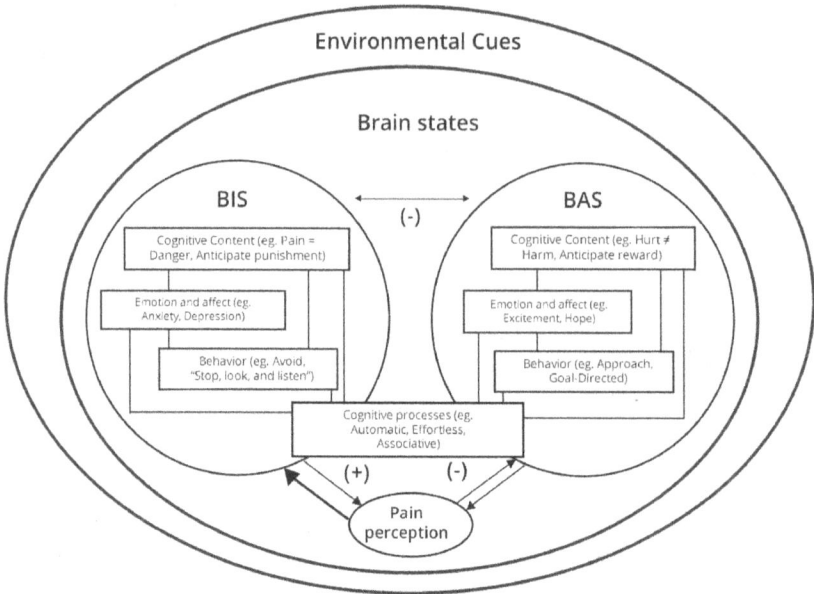

**Figure 16. BIS-BAS model of chronic pain**. Reprinted with permission from publisher from Jensen MP, Ehde DM, Day MA. The behavioral activation and inhibition systems: implications for understanding and treating chronic pain. J Pain.(18)

The BIS is sensitive to cues of danger and punishment, detecting threatening stimuli or events and promoting avoidance behaviors.(14),(18). The BAS is sensitive to cues of reward and encourages approach behaviors.(14),(18) Different types of BIS-BAS sensitivity are linked to different disorders. People with higher BIS sensitivity are prone to anxiety and depression, and tend to worry and ruminate.(14) Higher BIS scores are associated with higher levels of pain intensity,(14) greater pain interference, and less positive function.(19) People with high BAS sensitivity show greater positive function, despite pain, but are vulnerable to addiction disorders.(14),(19) Lower BAS scores are, for example, found in people suffering from fibromyalgia.(14) The BIS system is more dominant in the neurophysiology of pain since pain is usually perceived as a threatening stimulus.(14),(18) Indeed, pain catastrophizing, depression, anxiety, and pain-related avoidance behaviors are BIS-related features and are linked to maintenance of the threat value of the pain stimulus.(12)

Pain related-fear is strongly associated with perceived disability and reduced behavioral performance, even more strongly so than pain itself.(20) Patients scoring higher on pain catastrophizing and pain-related fear questionnaires show increased pain sensitivity.(21) Increased pain sensitivity is independently associated with self-reported avoidance, pain severity, functional avoidance, and self-reported disability.(21) Patients with chronic LBP, as well as pain-free individuals with higher scores on pain-related fear questionnaires, use less spinal flexion during lifting tasks, showing an unfavorable interaction between psychological factors and spinal motion.(5) Altered spinal motion, aimed at maintaining a protective trunk movement strategy, poses a risk for LBP due to pro-nociceptive inputs, potentially leading to increased loading on spinal tissues and increased pain sensitivity.(5) Pro-nociceptive inputs and increased pain sensitivity are central processes linked to the fear-avoidance model. Chronic low back patient observing back-straining exercises show increased brain signal activity in circuitry associated with salience, social cognition, and mentalizing.(22) A correlation between the fear-avoidance model, pain sensitivity, and brain activity is emerging and needs to be considered in patients with MSK disorders.

Altered lifting movement strategies in chronic LBP patients and pain-free individuals are an example of kinesiophobia. Kinesiophobia relates to the pain-related fear of movement believed to be damaging to the body. Kinesiophobia unfavorably influences treatment outcomes in patients with chronic spinal pain.(23) Kinesiophobia is associated with self-reported pain and disability in women with patellofemoral pain, while patellofemoral joint loading is not.(24) Patients with hip and knee osteoarthritis demonstrate higher levels of kinesiophobia. Functional outcomes and the active range of motion of a total knee replacement are negatively impacted by kinesiophobia.(25)

The Fear-Avoidance Components Scale (FACS) is a measurement questionnaire that encompasses cognitive, emotional, and behavioral components.(26) The FACS has been shown to be a psychometrically valid and reliable measure, with high internal consistency.(20) (See Appendix E: Pain Catastrophizing)

# References

1. Uritani D, Kasza J, Campbell PK, et al. The association between psychological characteristics and physical activity levels in people with knee osteoarthritis: a cross-sectional analysis. *BMC Musculoskelet Disord.* 2020;21:269. doi:10.1186/s12891-020-03305-2

2. Silbernagel KG, Hanlon S, Sprague A. Current clinical concepts: conservative management of achilles tendinopathy. *J Athl Train.* 2020;55(5):438-447. doi:10.4085/1062-6050-356-19

3. Lentz TA, George SZ, Manickas-Hill O, et al. What general and pain-associated psychological distress phenotypes exist among patients with hip and knee osteoarthritis? *Clin Orthop Relat Res.* 2020;478(12):2768-2783. doi:10.1097/corr.0000000000001520

4. Butera KA, Bishop MD, Greenfield WH 3rd, et al. Sensory and psychological factors predict exercise-induced shoulder injury responses in a high-risk phenotype cohort. *J Pain.* 2021;22(6):669-679. doi:10.1016/j.jpain.2020.12.002

5. Knechtle D, Schmid S, Suter M, et al. Fear-avoidance beliefs are associated with reduced lumbar spine flexion during object lifting in pain-free adults. *Pain.* 2021;162(6):1621-1631. doi:10.1097/j.pain.0000000000002170

6. Matheve T, De Baets L, Bogaerts K, et al. Lumbar range of motion in chronic low back pain is predicted by task-specific, but not by general measures of pain-related fear. *Eur J Pain.* 2019;23(6):1171-1184. doi:10.1002/ejp.1384

7. Ranger TA, Cicuttini FM, Jensen TS, et al. Catastrophization, fear of movement, anxiety, and depression are associated with persistent, severe low back pain and disability. *Spine J.* 2020;20(6):857-865. doi:10.1016/j.spinee.2020.02.002

8. De Baets L, Matheve T, Timmermans A. The association between fear of movement, pain catastrophizing, pain anxiety, and protective motor behavior in persons with peripheral joint conditions of a musculoskeletal origin: a systematic review. *Am J Phys Med Rehabil.* 2020;99(10):941-949. doi:10.1097/phm.0000000000001455

9. Vlaeyen JWS, Linton SJ. Fear-avoidance and its consequences in chronic musculoskeletal pain: a state of the art. *Pain.* 2000;85(3):317-332. doi:10.1016/S0304-3959(99)00242-0

10. Vlaeyen JWS, Crombez G, Linton SJ. The fear-avoidance model of pain. *Pain.* 2016;157(8):1588-1589. doi:10.1097/j.pain.0000000000000574

11. Bunzli S, Smith A, Schütze R, et al. Making sense of low back pain and pain-related fear. *J Orthop Sports Phys Ther.* 2017;47(9):628-636. doi:10.2519/jospt.2017.7434

12. van Vliet CM, Meulders A, Vancleef LMG, et al. The opportunity to avoid pain may paradoxically increase fear. *J Pain.* 2018;19(10):1222-1230. doi:10.1016/j.jpain.2018.05.003

13. van Vliet CM, Meulders A, Vancleef LMG, Vlaeyen JWS. Avoidance behaviour performed in the context of a novel, ambiguous movement increases threat and pain-related fear. *Pain.* 2021;162(3):875-885. doi:10.1097/j.pain.0000000000002079

14. Petrini L, Arendt-Nielsen L. Understanding pain catastrophizing: putting pieces together. *Front Psychol.* 2020;11:603420. doi:10.3389/fpsyg.2020.603420

15. Flink IL, Boersma K, Linton SJ. Pain catastrophizing as repetitive negative thinking: a development of the conceptualization. *Cogn Behav Ther.* 2013;42(3):215-223. doi:10.1080/16506073.2013.769621

16. Eccleston C, Crombez G. Worry and chronic pain: a misdirected problem solving model. *Pain.* 2007;132(3):233-236. doi:10.1016/j.pain.2007.09.014

17. Stroebe M, Boelen PA, van den Hout M, et al. Ruminative coping as avoidance: a reinterpretation of its function in adjustment to bereavement. *Eur Arch Psychiatry Clin Neurosci.* 2007;257(8):462-472. doi:10.1007/s00406-007-0746-y

18. Jensen MP, Ehde DM, Day MA. The behavioral activation and inhibition systems: implications for understanding and treating chronic pain. *J Pain.* 2016;17(5):529.e1-529.e18. doi:10.1016/j.jpain.2016.02.001

19. Turner AP, Jensen MP, Day MA, et al. Behavioral activation and behavioral inhibition: An examination of function in chronic pain. *Rehabil Psychol.* 2021;66(1):57-64. doi:10.1037/rep0000316

20. Gatchel RJ, Neblett R, Kishino N, et al. Fear-avoidance beliefs and chronic pain. *J Orthop Sports Phys Ther.* 2016;46(2):38-43. doi:10.2519/jospt.2016.0601

21. Uddin Z, Woznowski-Vu A, Flegg D, et al. Evaluating the novel added value of neurophysiological pain sensitivity within the fear-avoidance model of pain. *Eur J Pain.* 2019;23(5):957-972. doi:10.1002/ejp.1364

22. Ellingsen DM, Napadow V, Protsenko E, et al. Brain mechanisms of anticipated painful movements and their modulation by manual therapy in chronic low back pain. *J Pain.* 2018;19(11):1352-1365. doi:10.1016/j.jpain.2018.05.012

23. van Bogaert W, Coppieters I, Kregel J, et al. Influence of baseline kinesiophobia levels on treatment outcome in people with chronic spinal pain. *Phys Ther.* 2021;101(6):pzab076. doi:10.1093/ptj/pzab076

24. Silva DDO, Willy RW, Barton CJ, et al. Pain and disability in women with patellofemoral pain relate to kinesiophobia, but not to patellofemoral joint loading variables. *Scand J Med Sci Sports.* 2020;30(11):2215–2221. doi:10.1111/sms.13767

25. Brown OS, Hu L, Demetriou C, et al. The effects of kinesiophobia on outcome following total knee replacement: a systematic review. *Arch Orthop Trauma Surg.* 2020;140(12):2057-2070. doi:10.1007/s00402-020-03582-5

26. Neblett R, Mayer TG, Hartzell MM, et al. The fear-avoidance components scale (FACS): development and psychometric evaluation of a new measure of pain-related fear avoidance. *Pain Pract.* 2016;16(4):435-450. doi:10.1111/papr.12333

Michael Vianin MSc DC

# Depression

—⚯—

Depression, as described in the Pain Catastrophizing chapter, is linked to chronic pain, and associated with poorer outcomes and prognosis in MSK disorders. Evidence suggests that pain and depression share common pathophysiological pathways and have a reciprocal relationship.(1) Shared pathophysiological characteristics include cortical processing, immune mechanisms, and neurophysiological mechanisms.(1),(2),(3),(4),(5),(6) Persistent pain symptoms prevent depressed people from gaining better social and professional function, while depression increases the severity and distress associated with pain.(1) Pain and depression show overlapping changes in blood flow and neurotransmitters, in areas of the pain matrix.(3) Similar morphological and functional changes in brain regions and circuits have been found in both conditions.(3),(5) The brain areas most commonly found to have gray matter volume loss and alterations in activity in both conditions are the prefrontal cortex, anterior cingulate cortex, nucleus accumbens, hippocampus, and amygdala.(5) Pro- and anti-inflammatory cytokines activity affects pain and depression in similar ways.(3),(6) Inflammation in the central nervous system contributes to pain sensitization and chronification.(4) Inflammatory processes in depression induce alteration in the immune regulation of the central nervous system, further enhancing the central inflammatory process.(4),(6) This feedback mechanism leads to increased pain and depression.(4) Inflammatory cytokines also negatively impact serotonin production and serotonergic neurotransmission. (6) Serotonin and other neurotransmitters such as substance P, glutamate, dopamine, and norepinephrine are involved in common neurobiological pathways for pain and depression, likely contributing to their coexistence. (2),(6) The periaqueductal gray relays signals from the limbic system to the brainstem.(2) Serotonergic and noradrenergic cells within the relay system modulate pain perception by suppressing incoming nociceptive information. (2) Serotonin and norepinephrine depletion, associated with depression and inflammation, leads to the loss of the suppressing modulatory effect from the relay system.(2) Nociception is increased, attention to pain is heightened, and affect is negatively altered.(2) Therefore, the association between pain and depression can be linked to a common descending pathway in the central nervous system.(2)

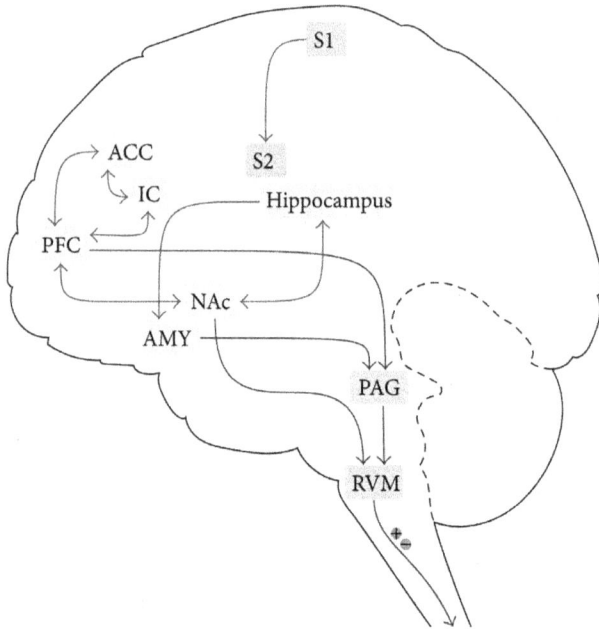

→ Descending pain modulation pathway.
— Circuits that modify depressive symptoms of pain.
●⊕ "on" cells in the RVM facilitate pain; "off" cells inhibit pain.
    Affective-motivational regions.
    Sensory-discriminative regions.

**Figure 17. Brain regions and circuits implicated in the comorbidity between pain and depression.** ACC = anterior cingulate cortex; AMY = amygdala; IC = insular cortex; NAc = nucleus accumbens; PAG = periaqueductal gray; PFC = prefrontal cortex; RVM = rostral ventromedial medulla; S1 = primary somatosensory cortex; S2 = secondary somatosensory cortex. Reprinted under the terms of the Creative Commons Attribution 3.0 International License from Doan L, Manders T, Wang J. Neuroplasticity underlying the comorbidity of pain and depression. Neural Plast.(5)

Pain and depression coexistence is explained, as described above, by shared anatomy and physiology. Patients suffering from chronic pain associated with MSK disorders are too often labeled as showing signs of somatization related to depressed mood or depression. The reciprocal relationship between pain and depression shows that such labeling is not only unhelpful but potentially harmful since the origin of either condition is dependent on their interplay. Given the close relationship between pain and depression, patients presenting with pain alone must be screened for depression and, conversely, patients presenting with depression alone need to be screened for pain.(7)

The Visual Analogue Scale, the Numeric Rating Scale, and the Verbal Rating Scale are quick and simple tools to use to assess pain.(7) The Brief Pain Inventory short form explores pain in more detail and shows high test-retest reliability.(7)

The National Institute for Health and Care Excellence (NICE) guideline screening for depression is a very brief, useful tool for a quick screening (see Appendix F: Depression).(7),(8) Well validated screening tools for depression include the short version of the Patient Health Questionnaire and the much more detailed Beck Depression Inventory.(7)

Management strategies for patients affected by MSK disorders should aim at understanding the unique contribution of depression to a patient's disposition and educate patients about the contribution of depression to their clinical presentation. Appropriate therapy should be offered if required.

# References

1. Rocca E, Anjum RL. Causal evidence and dispositions in medicine and public health. *Int J Environ Res Public Health*. 2020;17(6):1813. doi:10.3390/ijerph17061813

2. Michaelides A, Zis P. Depression, anxiety and acute pain: links and management challenges. *Postgrad Med*. 2019;131(7):438-444. doi:10.1080/00325481.2019.1663705

3. Gambassi G. Pain and depression: the egg and the chicken story revisited. *Arch Gerontol Geriatr*. 2009;49 (Suppl 1):103-112. doi:10.1016/j.archger.2009.09.018

4. Zis P, Daskalaki A, Bountouni I, et al. Depression and chronic pain in the elderly: links and management challenges. *Clin Interv Aging*. 2017;12:709-720. doi:10.2147/CIA.S113576

5. Doan L, Manders T, Wang J. Neuroplasticity underlying the comorbidity of pain and depression. *Neural Plast*. 2015;2015:a504691. doi:10.1155/2015/504691

6. Chimenti MS, Fonti GL, Conigliaro P, et al. The burden of depressive disorders in musculoskeletal diseases: is there an association between mood and inflammation? *Ann Gen Psychiatry*. 2021;20:1. doi:10.1186/s12991-020-00322-2

7. Cocksedge K, Shankar R, Simon C. Depression and pain: the need for a new screening tool. *Prog Neurol Psychiatry*. 2016;20:26–32. http://doi.wiley.com/10.1002/pnp.414

8. National Collaborating Centre for Mental Health (UK). *Depression in Adults with a Chronic Physical Health Problem: Treatment and Management.* Leicester, UK): British Psychological Society; 2010. (NICE Clinical Guidelines, No. 91.) Available from: https://www.ncbi.nlm.nih.gov/books/NBK82916/

# Sleep Quality

Lack of sleep is associated with increased pain perception and widespread pain. Insomnia promotes the transition from local pain to generalized pain in a dose-dependent manner.(1)

Sleep restriction is associated with poor cognitive performance and poor emotional regulation. It negatively impacts metabolism, immune, and cardiovascular functions, all of which are associated with increased pain sensitivity. Sleep deprivation increases pain responses and behaviors, exacerbates existing pain conditions, and reduces analgesic efficacy.(2),(3)

Pain stimulus can also disrupt sleep, but it mustn't be assumed that this is the case for every pain patient. More than 50% of chronic pain patients report poor sleep quality, the remaining chronic pain patients do not.(2)

Some sleep disorders (primary insomnia, narcolepsy, and restless leg syndrome) can also be associated with increased pain complaints in some, but not all, patients.(2)

Multiple pathways are involved in the development of sleep loss-induced hyperalgesia.

- The immune system is heavily involved in the development of pain by promoting inflammation and increasing nociceptor sensitivity. The immune system is, in turn, heavily regulated by circadian and sleep-wake cycles.(4) Lack of sleep is associated with increased numbers and enhanced activity of circulating leukocytes, especially neutrophils and monocytes. Increased monocyte activity leads to increased cytokines and C-reactive protein production, while increased neutrophil activation yields increased production of interleukins and prostaglandins. Overall, these changes promote inflammation, increase pronociceptive signaling and decrease antinociception.(2)

- Lack of sleep amplifies nociceptive inputs in the central nervous system (CNS) such as a gain in excitability of spinal nociceptive neurons, increased microglial activation, reduction of descending inhibitory controls, augmentation of excitatory descending pathways, loss of diffuse noxious inhibitory controls (DNICs), attenuation of positive affective pain inhibition, diminution of distraction analgesia, and reduction of placebo hypoalgesia.(2),(3)

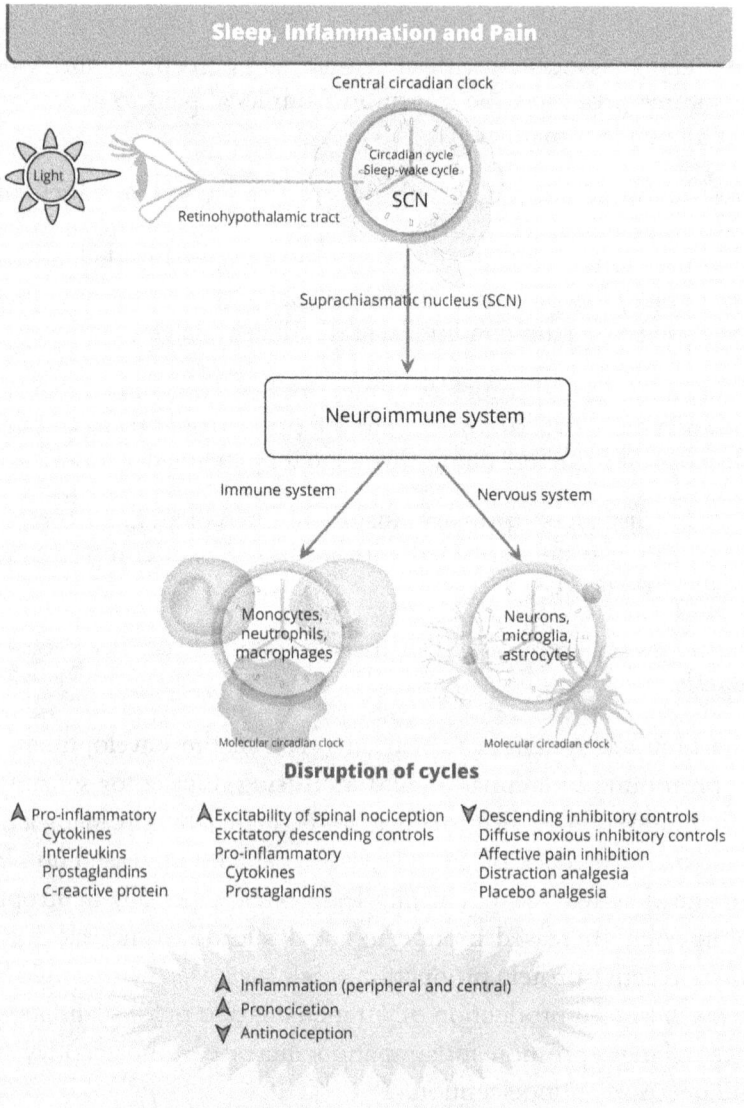

Figure 18. Sleep loss-induced inflammation and hyperalgesia.

Evaluation of insomnia symptoms and their causes must be part of the overall patient assessment. Strategies to improve sleep quality must be discussed and implemented with patients. The Pittsburgh Sleep Quality Index (PSQI) is a valid and reliable tool to measure sleep quality and patterns (see Appendix G: Sleep Quality).(5)

## References

1. Wiklund T, Gerdle B, Linton SJ, et al. Insomnia is a risk factor for spreading of chronic pain: a Swedish longitudinal population study (SwePain). *Eur J Pain*. 2020;24(7):1348-1356. doi:10.1002/ejp.1582

2. Alexandre C, Latremoliere A, Finan PH. Effect of Sleep Loss on Pain. *Oxford Handb Neurobiol Pain*. 2020;556–608. doi:10.1093/oxfordhb/9780190860509.013.31

3. Whibley D, AlKandari N, Kristensen K, et al. Sleep and Pain: A Systematic Review of Studies of Mediation. *Clin J Pain*. 2019;35(6):544-558. doi:10.1097/ajp.0000000000000697

4. Segal JP, Tresidder KA, Bhatt C, et al. Circadian control of pain and neuroinflammation. J Neurosci Res. 2018;96(6):1002-1020. doi:10.1002/jnr.24150

5. Mollayeva T, Thurairajah P, Burton K, et al. The Pittsburgh sleep quality index as a screening tool for sleep dysfunction in clinical and non-clinical samples: a systematic review and meta-analysis. *Sleep Med Rev*. 2016;25:52-73. doi:10.1016/j.smrv.2015.01.009

Michael Vianin MSc DC

# Metabolic Health

Chronic pain involves changes in neuronal structure, networks, and functions that promote amplification of pain perception.(1) Persistent low-grade inflammation (neuroinflammation) is a primary driver in this adaptive pain modulation.(1) Neuroinflammation is driven by neurotransmitters produced by neurons, and by neuroimmune mediators released by glial cells. (1),(2) The production and release of neurotransmitters and neuroimmune mediators are dependent on metabolic regulation.(3) Reduction in energy provision to neurons is potentially implicated in dysfunctions, such as Alzheimer's disease.(1),(4) Poor nutrition can result in glial activation, which can result in neuroimmune activation that ends up increasing inflammation and sensitization of the nervous system.(1),(5) Indeed, chronic metabolic diseases, such as obesity and diabetes are often comorbid with chronic pain. (1),(6),(7),(8) There is a definite link between chronic pain, inflammation, and metabolic regulation that needs to be assessed in patients affected by MSK disorders.

Accumulating evidence shows that pain and obesity are significantly related to each other.(7) Obese patients suffer more significantly from unrelieved chronic pain, leading to increased health care consumption and lower quality of life.(7),(9) Obesity is associated with various pain diagnoses, such as inflammatory forms of arthritis, osteoarthritis, low back pain, headaches, fibromyalgia, chronic widespread pain, pelvic pain, neuropathic pain, and abdominal pain.(7),(10),(11) Higher body mass index (BMI) is a persistent independent risk factor for back pain across adulthood.(12) Obesity is also associated with degenerative and inflammatory conditions of the MSK system.(13) Numerous studies show that obesity is related to the onset, progression and severity of osteoarthritis.(7),(10) Patients with a higher BMI, for example, have 35% increased risk of developing knee osteoarthritis.(14)

Conversely, weight gain may occur because of chronic pain. Other factors associated with chronic pain, including a sedentary lifestyle, poor sleep, and medication side-effects, contribute to weight gain in chronic pain patients.(7) Obese patients suffering from chronic pain have a greater physical disability and psychological distress than non-obese patients.(7) Frustration with functional limitations can lead to overeating and more weight gain.(7),(11)

Different mechanisms are involved in the obesity-pain association:

- **Mechanical stress:** the mechanical overloading on the musculoskeletal system is the most appraised link between obesity and pain. Weight surplus leads to increased mechanical stress that can contribute to pain.(7),(13),(15),(16) Sustained overloading on the MSK structure of the lower back, hip, and knee joints promotes the development of osteoarthritis and altered biomechanics, such as abnormal gait in obese patients.(7),(17) Increased mechanical loading prompts the degradation of Type II collagen, joint extracellular matrix, and hyaluronic acid fragmentation.(15) These factors, in turn, cause imbalance between deterioration and repair of the cartilage, chondrocyte apoptosis, reduced synovial fluid viscosity, and increased joint friction — all of which lead to changes in posture and movement and increasing pain scores.(15)

- **Inflammation:** the higher central adiposity associated with obesity is related to inflammatory processes due to increased body fat mass. Increased fat mass is recognized as a low-grade inflammatory disease and is linked to chronic pain.(10),(15),(16) Adipose tissue in obese individuals (white fat) contains adipocytes and pro-inflammatory immunocytes such as neutrophils, macrophages, innate lymphoid cells, T-cells, and B-cells.(10),(15) The number of circulating macrophages, monocytes, and neutrophils increases during obesity.(15)

  The adipose tissue inflammation is initiated by macrophages, but other immune cells also play a key role.(15) In adipose tissue, macrophages are activated into a pro-inflammatory macrophage type (M1), while in thin individuals, they are activated into an anti-inflammatory type (M2).(10),(15) The activated macrophages in obesity (M1) produce pro-inflammatory cytokines (e.g. interleukine-1-beta and interleukine-6, serum tumor necrosis factor-alpha) that sustain a constant low-grade inflammation and promote insulin resistance.(15)

  The T-cell subsets found in adipose tissue in obesity play a role in the transformation of macrophages into their pro-inflammatory form (M1).(10) B-cells are involved in the obesity-induced adipose tissue inflammation by stimulating T-cells and activating macrophages.(10)

Pro-inflammatory cytokines released by adipose tissue regulate the proliferation and apoptosis of adipocytes.(10) The apoptosis of adipocytes leads to the release of more cytokines and creates more systemic inflammation.(15) In addition, adipocytes tend to rupture in obese patients, leading to massive cellular apoptosis, which considerably increases the release of cytokines and leads to more inflammation.(15)

Excess fat is associated with increased secretion of inflammatory cytokines into the systemic circulation, as evidenced by higher levels of circulating interleukine-6, serum tumor necrosis factor-alpha, and C-reactive protein found in overweight and obese patients.(10) Higher levels of circulating interleukine-6, serum tumor necrosis factor-alpha, and C-reactive protein are associated with decreased muscle mass and muscle strength.(18)

Adipocytes are a major neuroendocrine organ that continually and systemically release pro-inflammatory factors, such as cytokines, chemokines, and metabolically-active adipokines.(7),(10),(15) Chemokines released by adipocytes activate the differentiation of monocytes into pro-inflammatory macrophages (M1),(15) which produce more pro-inflammatory cytokines.

Adipokines, such as adiponectin and leptin, regulate the inflammatory response in cartilage.(10) The circulating and cartilage levels of adipokines are increased in obesity.(15) Adipokines activate chondrocytes to secrete proteinases (matrix metalloproteinases), nitric oxide, and cytokines (interleukine-1-beta, interleukine-6, interleukine-8, and serum tumor necrosis factor-alpha). These mediators increase synovial inflammation and pain hypersensitivity,(15) and activate the production of more cytokines (proteinases and prostaglandins) that inhibit the production of proteoglycans and Type II collagen, and play a critical role in cartilage matrix degradation and bone resorption in osteoarthritis.(10)

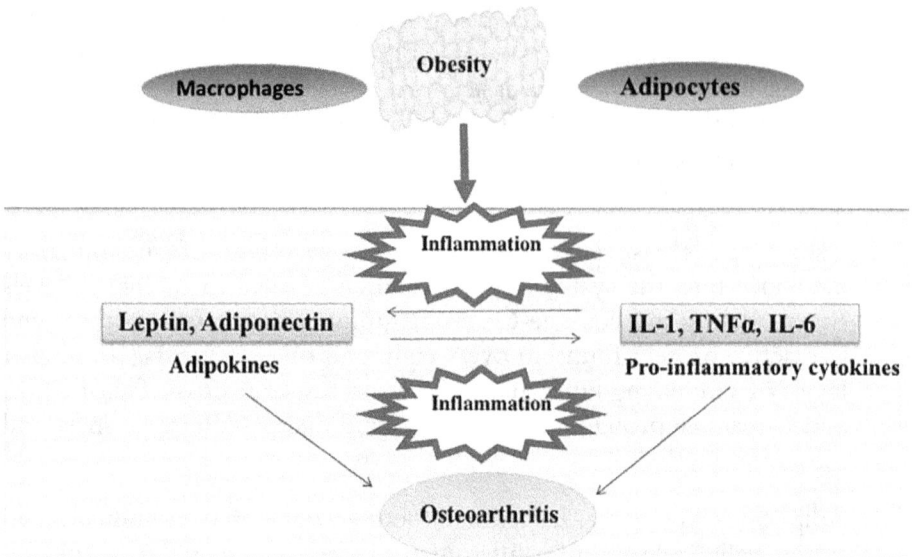

**Figure 19. The link between obesity and osteoarthritis.** In obese subjects, adipocytes and macrophages are the main source of an increased synthesis and secretion of adipcytokines (leptin, adiponectin) and pro-inflammatory cytokines (IL-1, TNFα, IL-6). Both adipcytokines and pro-inflammatory cytokines, can result in osteoarthritis. Reprinted with permission from publisher from Wang T, He C. Pro-inflammatory cytokines: the link between obesity and osteoarthritis. Cytokine Growth Factor Rev.(10)

- **Neuro-immunity**: peripheral immune activation modulates the development and the function of central pain pathways.(19) The sensory nervous system and the immune system work together to protect their host from threat, but they can also drive diseases (autoimmune disease, allergic reactions).(15) Nociceptors found in lymphoid tissues and in the mucosal barrier, interact with immune cells by releasing local neuropeptides.(15) Neurogenic inflammation promotes the secretion of peptides that influence inflammation.(15) For example, substance P promotes T-cell activity and increases dendritic cell recruitment, which leads to increased inflammation.(15) Adipose tissue in obesity releases local neuropeptides that will increase the number and the polarization of immune cells within the tissue, further increasing inflammation and nociceptor sensitivity.(15) Fat pads are often hyper-innervated and rich in immunocytes that also release cytokines, amplifying nociceptor function. Amplified nociception, in turn, sustains the function of immunocytes through the release of neuropeptides, creating a self-maintaining positive nociceptive feedback loop, which leads to nociceptor hypersensitivity and pain.(15) Nociceptor hypersensitivity, with time, can lead to peripheral and central neuroinflammation from glia activation.(20) Neuroinflammation results from glia activation in the peripheral nervous system (Schwann cells and satellite glial cells), and central nervous system (microglia and astrocytes), as well as from the activation and infiltration of immune cells (e.g. macrophages and T-cells).(20) Neuroinflammation in the peripheral nervous systems results in peripheral sensitization.(20) Alterations in the central nervous system, mediated by the enhancement of pain processing in the spinal cord and brain, lead to central sensitization, and widespread chronic pain.(20) Therefore, bidirectional signaling between the immune and nervous systems contributes to the development and maintenance of chronic pain.(20)

- **Psychological factors:** obese pain patients tend to have a greater fear of movement than non-obese pain patients.(7) Fear of movement (kinesiophobia) significantly contributes to pain and disability in MSK disorders (see chapter: Pain Catastrophizing). Such fear can lead to inactivity and physical deconditioning in obese patients, which, in turn, negatively impacts pain and weight.(7) Depression is another disposition associated with both pain and obesity. Depression is linked to chronic pain and is associated with poorer outcomes and prognosis in MSK disorders (see chapter: Depression). Depression can impact pain and obesity, as depression is associated with emotional eating and cravings for high-calorie comfort foods.(7) Low self-efficacy is another theme that links pain and obesity.(11) Obese pain patients report difficulties in completing simple, everyday tasks and feel discouraged by their limited level of activity.(11) They also become disinterested in attending active rehabilitation treatment strategies, because of the exacerbation in pain felt during their treatment, and because of the difficulties of exercising due to their comorbidity, particularly their limited mobility and low cardiovascular fitness.(11)

- **Sleep:** poor sleep is common in chronic pain patients and plays an important role in the inflammatory process (see chapter: Sleep Quality). Obese patients are more affected by sleep disturbance and, therefore, are more likely to show increased pain perception and widespread pain. (7),(21)

Diabetic patients have a significantly higher prevalence of chronic pain.(22) Chronic pain symptoms with higher prevalence in diabetic patients include lower limb pain, back pain, abdominal pain, and neck pain.(16), (22) Diabetes mellitus is an independent risk factor for chronic back pain (spinal pain, neck pain, or low back pain).(8),(23),(24) Numerous studies have shown a link between hyperglycemia and altered fat metabolism commonly present in diabetes, and vertebral degeneration and intervertebral disc degeneration, providing a potential mechanism by which diabetes can contribute to chronic back pain.(8),(23),(24) Chronic uncontrolled diabetes is linked to a higher likelihood of chronic low back pain and the development of spinal stenosis.(8) The association between diabetes and chronic back pain tends to be stronger for severe cases of chronic pain.(24)

Clinicians caring for patients with MSK disorders have to consider the status of a patient's metabolic health. Patients presenting with metabolic health dispositions that can negatively impact their condition, need to be educated about the link between their metabolic health status and their pain condition. Management strategies to positively impact their metabolic health need to be discussed and implemented to increase the chance of positive management outcomes.

# References

1. Field R, Pourkazemi F, Turton J, et al. Dietary interventions are beneficial for patients with chronic pain: a systematic review with meta-analysis. *Pain Med.* 2021;22(3):694-714. doi:10.1093/pm/pnaa378

2. Grace PM, Hutchinson MR, Maier SF, et al. Pathological pain and the neuroimmune interface. *Nat Rev Immunol.* 2014;14(4):217-231. doi:10.1038/nri3621

3. Jha MK, Morrison BM. Glia-neuron energy metabolism in health and diseases: new insights into the role of nervous system metabolic transporters. *Exp Neurol.* 2018;309:23-31. doi:10.1016/j.expneurol.2018.07.009

4. An Y, Varma VR, Varma S, et al. Evidence for brain glucose dysregulation in Alzheimer's disease. *Alzheimers Dement.* 2018;14(3):318-329. doi:10.1016/j.jalz.2017.09.011

5. Totsch SK, Waite ME, Sorge RE. Dietary influence on pain via the immune system. *Prog Mol Biol Transl Sci.* 2015;131:435-469. doi:10.1016/bs.pmbts.2014.11.013

6. Emery CF, Olson KL, Bodine A, et al. Dietary intake mediates the relationship of body fat to pain. *Pain.* 2017;158(2):273-277. doi:10.1097/j.pain.0000000000000754

7. Okifuji A, Hare BD. The association between chronic pain and obesity. *J Pain Res.* 2015;8:399-408. doi:10.2147/JPR.S55598

8. Rinaldo L, McCutcheon BA, Gilder H, et al. Diabetes and back pain: markers of diabetes disease progression are associated with chronic back pain. *Clin Diabetes.* 2017;35(3):126-131. doi:10.2337/cd16-0011

9. Thomazeau J, Perin J, Nizard R, et al. Pain management and pain characteristics in obese and normal weight patients before joint replacement. *J Eval Clin Pract.* 2014;20(5):611-616. doi:10.1111/jep.12176

10. Wang T, He C. Pro-inflammatory cytokines: the link between obesity and osteoarthritis. *Cytokine Growth Factor Rev.* 2018;44:38-50. doi:10.1016/j.cytogfr.2018.10.002

11. Janke EA, Kozak AT. "The more pain I have, the more I want to eat": obesity in the context of chronic pain. *Obesity (Silver Spring).* 2012;20(10):2027-2034. doi:10.1038/oby.2012.39

12. Muthuri S, Cooper R, Kuh D, et al. Do the associations of body mass index and waist circumference with back pain change as people age? 32 years of follow-up in a British birth cohort. *BMJ Open.* 2020;10(12):e039197. doi:10.1136/bmjopen-2020-039197

13. Anandacoomarasamy A, Fransen M, March L. Obesity and the musculoskeletal system. *Curr Opin Rheumatol.* 2009;21:71-77. doi:10.1097/bor.0b013e32831bc0d7

14. Jiang L, Tian W, Wang Y, et al. Body mass index and susceptibility to knee osteoarthritis: a systematic review and meta-analysis. *Joint Bone Spine.* 2012;79(3):291-297. doi:10.1016/j.jbspin.2011.05.015

15. Eichwald T, Talbot S. Neuro-immunity controls obesity-induced pain. *Front Hum Neurosci.* 2020;14:181. doi:10.3389/fnhum.2020.00181

16. Pozzobon D, Ferreira PH, Dario AB, et al. Is there an association between diabetes and neck and back pain? A systematic review with meta-analyses. *PLoS One.* 2019;14(2):e0212030. doi:10.1371/journal.pone.0212030

17. King LK, March L, Anandacoomarasamy A. Obesity & osteoarthritis. *Indian J Med Res.* 2013;138(2):185-193.

18. Tuttle CS, Thang LA, Maier AB. Markers of inflammation and their association with muscle strength and mass: a systematic review and meta-analysis. *Ageing Res Rev.* 2020;64:101185. doi:10.1016/j.arr.2020.101185

19. Karshikoff B, Tadros MA, Mackey S, et al. Neuroimmune modulation of pain across the developmental spectrum. *Curr Opin Behav Sci.* 2019;28:85-92. doi:10.1016/j.cobeha.2019.01.010

20. Buchheit T, Huh Y, Maixner W, et al. Neuroimmune modulation of pain and regenerative pain medicine. *J Clin Invest.* 2020;130(5):2164-2176. doi:10.1172/JCI134439

21. Wiklund T, Gerdle B, Linton SJ, et al. Insomnia is a risk factor for spreading of chronic pain: a Swedish longitudinal population study (SwePain). *Eur J Pain.* 2020;24(7):1348-1356. doi:10.1002/ejp.1582

22. Aldossari KK, Shubair MM, Al-Zahrani J, et al. Association between chronic pain and diabetes/prediabetes: a population-based cross-sectional survey in Saudi Arabia. *Pain Res Manag.* 2020;2020:8239474. doi:10.1155/2020/8239474

23. Pico-Espinosa OJ, Skillgate E, Tettamanti G, et al. Diabetes mellitus and hyperlipidaemia as risk factors for frequent pain in the back, neck and/or shoulders/arms among adults in Stockholm 2006 to 2010 - results from the Stockholm Public Health Cohort. *Scand J Pain.* 2017;15:1-7. doi:10.1016/j.sjpain.2016.11.005

24. Dario A, Ferreira M, Refshauge K, et al. Mapping the association between back pain and type 2 diabetes: a cross-sectional and longitudinal study of adult Spanish twins. *PLoS One.* 2017;12(4):e0174757. doi:10.1371/journal.pone.0174757

# Physical Activity

The World Health Organization (WHO) declared insufficient physical activity as a leading risk factor for non-communicable diseases and death worldwide.(1) Sedentary behavior is damaging to health, physical function, and health-related quality of life.(1) Prolonged, continuous sedentary behavior is associated with pain and disability, as each additional daily hour of sedentary behavior has been reported to result in 46% greater odds of disability with activities of daily living.(1)

On the other hand, physical activity and/or physical exercise show a positive correlation with health benefits.(2) Health benefits derived from physical activity include enhanced musculoskeletal function, cardiorespiratory and metabolic health, sleep, pain management, cognition, learning, and memory.(2) Physical activity is a well-documented treatment for chronic pain conditions with beneficial effects on pain, sleep, cognitive function, and physical function.(1) Growing evidence shows physical activity as beneficial for many chronic illnesses, including cardiovascular disease, Type 2 diabetes, and obesity.(1) Physical activity has a positive impact on quality of life, activities of daily living, emotional affect, overall physical function, and independence.(1) Regular physical activity is a significant tool for both primary and secondary prevention of chronic disease with the ability to alleviate symptoms and slow or stop disease progression.(1) Recent studies show that staying or becoming active and exercising are central to MSK rehabilitation.(3),(4),(5)

Proposed mechanisms of action in MSK rehabilitation are neuromuscular, psychosocial, neurophysiological, cardiometabolic, immunological, and tissue healing.(2),(6),(7).

- Neuromuscular mechanisms include improved muscular strength, power, and endurance; increased flexibility of soft tissue, and improved motor control.(6),(7)

- Psychosocial mechanisms consist of improvements in fear-avoidance, pain self-efficacy, mood, disability perception, social support, catastrophizing, and kinesiophobia.(6),(7),(8),(9)

- Physical activity and exercise can reduce pain sensitivity and induce hypoalgesia.(10),(11),(12) Neurophysiological mechanisms involved are secretion of endorphins, activation of descending inhibition and gate control, improvement in stress response, increase in pain threshold, increased cerebral perfusion, and promotion of central neuroplastic changes .(6),(7),(10),(13),(14) Regular exercise alters central facilitation by decreasing descending facilitation, resulting in a net increase in inhibition.(15) Physical activity also reduces spinal nociception by increasing nociceptive flexion reflex threshold.(16)

- Cardiometabolic mechanisms entail an improvement in aerobic fitness, body composition, and body weight; and prevention of comorbidity (cardiovascular diseases, respiratory diseases, and diabetes mellitus). (6),(7)

- Modulation of the immune system is involved in the beneficial effect of exercise in MSK care. Regular practice of moderate-intensity physical exercise directs the immune system to an anti-inflammatory response. (2) The beneficial effects of physical exercise on the inflammatory response and health outcomes are intensity dependent.(2) Regular moderate exercise intensity, yields the best response and outcomes (see Appendix H: Physical Activity).(2)

- Tissue healing mechanisms comprise increased blood flow; decreased inflammation; modulation of bone, ligaments, tendons, and cartilage; and tissue restoration.(6),(7)

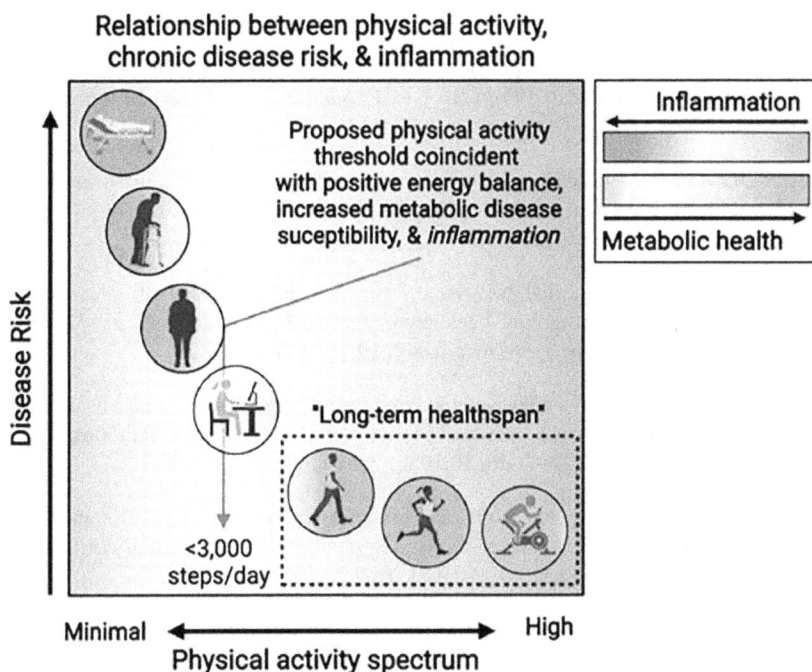

**Fig 20. Relationship between physical activity, chronic disease, and inflammation.** Maintaining adequate physical activity levels is necessary to increase health span. Physical inactivity is a contributor to multiple pathological conditions and is now highlighted as a leading cause of death in Western societies. Present data suggest that a causative activity threshold (<3,000 steps per day) exists, whereby dipping below this level of activity may evoke insulin resistance and increase the likelihood of positive energy balance. Emerging data also reveal that periods of physical inactivity provoke inflammatory signaling in various tissues and cell types; however, whether a similar activity threshold exists for inflammatory-based diseases as insulin resistance is currently unknown. Reprinted with permission from publisher from Winn, N.C., Cottam, M.A., Wasserman, D.H. and Hasty, A.H. Exercise and Adipose Tissue Immunity: Outrunning Inflammation. Obesity.(17)

The level of physical activity needs to be discussed with patients suffering from MSK disorders. Exercise recommendations must be considered in collaboration with patients. Regular moderate-intensity exercise enhances the immune function response, reinforces the antioxidative capacity, reduces oxidative stress, and increases the efficiency of energy generation, therefore reducing the incidence of inflammatory diseases.(2) Increased physical activity is associated with better subjective sleep quantity and quality.(18) The type of exercise does not seem to matter as much as doing some form of physical activity.(19),(20) Therefore, clinicians need to promote regular moderate-intensity exercise by finding activities that are meaningful, achievable, and enjoyable for patients.(21),(22)

109

# References

1. Ambrose KR, Golightly YM. Physical exercise as non-pharmacological treatment of chronic pain: why and when. *Best Pract Res Clin Rheumatol.* 2015;29:120-130. doi:10.1016/j.berh.2015.04.022

2. Scheffer DD, Latini A. Exercise-induced immune system response: anti-inflammatory status on peripheral and central organs. *Biochim Biophys Acta Mol Basis Dis.* 2020;1866(10):165823. doi:10.1016/j.bbadis.2020.165823

3. Owen PJ, Miller CT, Mundell NL, et al. Which specific modes of exercise training are most effective for treating low back pain? Network meta-analysis. *Br J Sports Med.* 2020;54(21):1279-1287. doi:10.1136/bjsports-2019-100886

4. de Zoete RM, Brown L, Oliveira K, et al. The effectiveness of general physical exercise for individuals with chronic neck pain: a systematic review of randomised controlled trials. *Eur. J. Physiother.* 2019;22(3):141–7. doi:10.1080/21679169.2018.1561942

5. Bricca A, Harris LK, Jäger M, et al. Benefits and harms of exercise therapy in people with multimorbidity: a systematic review and meta-analysis of randomised controlled trials. *Ageing Res Rev.* 2020;63:101166. doi:10.1016/j.arr.2020.101166

6. Wun A, Kollias P, Jeong H, et al. Why is exercise prescribed for people with chronic low back pain? A review of the mechanisms of benefit proposed by clinical trialists. *Musculoskelet Sci Pract.* 2021;51:102307. doi:10.1016/j.msksp.2020.102307

7. Beckwée D, Vaes P, Cnudde M, et al. Osteoarthritis of the knee: why does exercise work? A qualitative study of the literature. *Ageing Res Rev.* 2013;12:226-236. doi:10.1016/j.arr.2012.09.005

8. Hanel J, Owen PJ, Held S, et al. Effects of exercise training on fear-avoidance in pain and pain-free populations: systematic review and meta-analysis. *Sports Med.* 2020;50(12):2193-2207. doi:10.1007/s40279-020-01345-1

9. Izquierdo-Alventosa R, Inglés M, Cortés-Amador S, et al. Low-intensity physical exercise improves pain catastrophizing and other psychological and physical aspects in women with fibromyalgia: a randomized controlled trial. *Int J Environ Res Public Health.* 2020;17(10):3634. doi:10.3390/ijerph17103634

10. Belavy DL, Van Oosterwijck J, Clarkson M, et al. Pain sensitivity is reduced by exercise training: evidence from a systematic review and meta-analysis. *Neurosci Biobehav Rev.* 2021;120:100-108. doi:10.1016/j.neubiorev.2020.11.012

11. Wewege MA, Jones MD. Exercise-induced hypoalgesia in healthy individuals and people with chronic musculoskeletal pain: a systematic review and meta-analysis. *J Pain.* 2021;22:21-31. doi:10.1016/j.jpain.2020.04.003

12. Guzmán-Pavón MJ, Cavero-Redondo I, Martínez-Vizcaíno V, et al. Effect of physical exercise programs on myofascial trigger points-related dysfunctions: a systematic review and meta-analysis. *Pain Med.* 2020;21(11):2986-2996. doi:10.1093/pm/pnaa253

13. Hansen S, Dalgaard RC, Mikkelsen PS, et al. Modulation of exercise-induced hypoalgesia following an exercise intervention in healthy subjects. *Pain Med.* 2020;21(12):3556-3566. doi:10.1093/pm/pnaa212

14. Vaegter HB, Jones MD. Exercise-induced hypoalgesia after acute and regular exercise: experimental and clinical manifestations and possible mechanisms in individuals with and without pain. *Pain Rep.* 2020;5(5):e823. doi:10.1097/pr9.0000000000000823

15. Sluka KA, Danielson J, Rasmussen L, et al. Regular physical activity reduces the percentage of spinally projecting neurons that express mu-opioid receptors from the rostral ventromedial medulla in mice. *Pain Rep.* 2020;5(6):e857. doi:10.1097/pr9.0000000000000857

16. Dhondt E, Danneels L, van Oosterwijck S, et al. The influence of physical activity on the nociceptive flexion reflex in healthy people. *Eur J Pain.* 2021;25(4):774-789. doi:10.1002/ejp.1708

17. Winn, N.C., Cottam, M.A., Wasserman, D.H. and Hasty, A.H. Exercise and Adipose Tissue Immunity: Outrunning Inflammation. *Obesity.* 2021;29:790-801. doi:10.1002/oby.23147

18. Mochón-Benguigui S, Carneiro-Barrera A, Castillo MJ, et al. Role of physical activity and fitness on sleep in sedentary middle-aged adults: the FIT-AGEING study. *Sci Rep.* 2021;11:539. doi:10.1038/s41598-020-79355-2

19. Ferro Moura Franco K, Lenoir D, Dos Santos Franco YR, et al. Prescription of exercises for the treatment of chronic pain along the continuum of nociplastic pain: a systematic review with meta-analysis. *Eur J Pain.* 2021;25:51-70. doi:10.1002/ejp.1666

20. Vanti C, Andreatta S, Borghi S, et al. The effectiveness of walking versus exercise on pain and function in chronic low back pain: a systematic review and meta-analysis of randomized trials. *Disabil Rehabil.* 2019;41(6):622-632. doi:10.1080/09638288.2017.1410730

21. Ferreira GE, Howard K, Zadro JR, et al. People considering exercise to prevent low back pain recurrence prefer exercise programs that differ from programs known to be effective: a discrete choice experiment. *J Physiother.* 2020;66(4):249-255. doi:10.1016/j.jphys.2020.09.011

22. Thompson WR, Sallis R, Joy E, et al. Exercise Is Medicine. *Am. J. Lifestyle Med.* 2020;14(5):511-523. doi:10.1177/1559827620912192

Michael Vianin MSc DC

# Self-Efficacy

———∞———

Self-efficacy, the belief in one's ability to manage and complete a task despite pain, is associated with lower disability, less pain, reduced disease activity, fewer depressive symptoms, less fatigue, less fear and emotional distress, greater adherence to physical activity, and improved quality of life in people suffering from chronic musculoskeletal pain.[1],[2],[3],[4] Self-efficacy determines how much effort and persistence a patient with an MSK disorder demonstrates when facing obstacles or difficult experiences,[3] and includes self-confidence, accurate self-evaluation, a willingness to take risks, and a sense of accomplishment.[4] In the rehabilitation of MSK disorders, self-efficacy facilitates activity participation and moderates treatment response. [1],[2],[5],[6],[7] Self-efficacy influences pain and associated outcomes by helping patients accomplish necessary actions to manage and control pain itself.[3] Furthermore, perceived self-efficacy determines the way in which pain is dealt with in specific situations.[3] For example, a patient with low self-efficacy will avoid activities that create pain, or take more pain medication in such situations; while a patient with high self-efficacy will engage in new challenges, despite pain.[3] The sense of self-efficacy will be further diminished in a patient with low baseline self-efficacy, because of the lack of success in controlling painful activities.[3] Inversely, a patient with high self-efficacy will be comforted in their capacity to deal with painful situations and to master new activities, despite pain, which, in turn, will increase their sense of self-efficacy.[3]

Low self-efficacy is comorbidly associated with other pain-promoting dispositions, including longer pain duration, older age (see chapter: Social Determinants of Health), belonging to certain ethnic groups (see chapter: Culture), depressive symptoms (see chapter: Depression), health literacy (see chapter: Health Literacy), and obesity (see chapter: Metabolic Health). [3],[4],[8],[9],[10]

The assessment of self-efficacy in patients affected by MSK disorders is fundamental, in order to establish a comprehensive rehabilitation program. The most widely used instruments are the Pain Self-Efficacy Questionnaire and the Chronic Pain Self-Efficacy Scale,(11) and both are suitable for the chronic pain population in general.(12) The Pain Self-Efficacy Questionnaire only addresses the confidence to maintain everyday life, while the Chronic Pain Self-Efficacy Scale addresses beliefs about the ability to control pain, negative emotions associated with pain, and the ability to maintain everyday life activities, including work.(12) The Chronic Pain Self-Efficacy Scale is more encompassing and better suited to get a general idea of a patient's self-efficacy (see Appendix I: Self-Efficacy).

Patients suffering from MSK disorders need to be educated about self-efficacy and its impact on symptom management. In patients demonstrating low self-efficacy, strategies to improve self-efficacy (e.g. graded activity, behavioral counseling), need to be discussed and implemented to achieve a better treatment response.(1),(3),(4),(5),(13)

## References

1. Martinez-Calderon J, Flores-Cortes M, Morales-Asencio JM, et al. Which interventions enhance pain self-efficacy in people with chronic musculoskeletal pain? A systematic review with meta-analysis of randomized controlled trials, including over 12,000 participants. *J Orthop Sports Phys Ther.* 2020;50(8):418-430. doi:10.2519/jospt.2020.9319

2. De Baets L, Matheve T, Meeus M, et al. The influence of cognitions, emotions and behavioral factors on treatment outcomes in musculoskeletal shoulder pain: a systematic review. *Clin Rehabil.* 2019;33(6):980-991. doi:10.1177/0269215519831056

3. Jackson T, Wang Y, Wang Y, et al. Self-efficacy and chronic pain outcomes: a meta-analytic review. *J Pain.* 2014;15(8):800-814. doi:10.1016/j.jpain.2014.05.002

4. Martinez-Calderon J, Zamora-Campos C, Navarro-Ledesma S, et al. The role of self-efficacy on the prognosis of chronic musculoskeletal pain: a systematic review. *J Pain.* 2018;19:10-34. doi:10.1016/j.jpain.2017.08.008

5. Martin ES, Dobson F, Hall M, et al. The effects of behavioural counselling on the determinants of health behaviour change in adults with chronic musculoskeletal conditions making lifestyle changes: a systematic review and meta-analysis. *Musculoskeletal Care.* 2019;17(3):170-197. doi:10.1002/msc.1410

6. Hayward R, Stynes S. Self-efficacy as a prognostic factor and treatment moderator in chronic musculoskeletal pain patients attending pain management programmes: a systematic review. *Musculoskeletal Care.* 2020;10.1002/msc.1533. doi:10.1002/msc.1533

7. Christe G, Nzamba J, Desarzens L, et al. Physiotherapists' attitudes and beliefs about low back pain influence their clinical decisions and advice. *Musculoskelet Sci Pract.* 2021;53:102382. doi:10.1016/j.msksp.2021.102382

8. Orhan C, Van Looveren E, Cagnie B, et al. Are pain beliefs, cognitions, and behaviors influenced by race, ethnicity, and culture in patients with chronic musculoskeletal pain: a systematic review. *Pain Physician*. 2018;21(6):541-558.

9. Ferreira-Valente MA, Pais-Ribeiro JL, Jensen MP. Associations between psychosocial factors and pain intensity, physical functioning, and psychological functioning in patients with chronic pain: a cross-cultural comparison. *Clin J Pain*. 2014;30(8):713-723. doi:10.1097/ajp.0000000000000027

10. Kapoor S, Eyer J, Thorn B. Health literacy in individuals with chronic pain living in rural United States: association with pain-related variables. *J Pain*. 2016;17(4):S17–S18. doi:10.1016/j.jpain.2016.01.071

11. Vergeld V, Utesch T. Pain-related self-efficacy among people with back pain: a systematic review of assessment tools. *Clin J Pain*. 2020; 36(6):480–494. doi:10.1097/ajp.0000000000000818

12. Miles CL, Pincus T, Carnes D, et al. Measuring pain self-efficacy. *Clin J Pain*. 2011;27(5):461-470. doi:10.1097/ajp.0b013e318208c8a2

13. Williamson W, Kluzek S, Roberts N, et al. Behavioural physical activity interventions in participants with lower-limb osteoarthritis: a systematic review with meta-analysis. *BMJ Open*. 2015;5(8):e007642. doi:10.1136/bmjopen-2015-007642

# Locus of Control

Health locus of control refers to the representation of the extent to which individuals take control of, and responsibility for, their health (internal locus), as opposed to environmental factors, chance, luck, fate, or powerful others (external locus).(1),(2),(3),(4) An internal health locus of control is the belief that individuals themselves are responsible for their conditions. An external health locus of control is the belief that the responsibility for a condition can be attributed to factors outside the realm of one's control.(1),(2),(3),(4)

Patients with MSK disorders, who have a high external locus of control, have more disability, increased psychological issues, increased use of health care services, negative coping strategies, increased drug abuse, and decreased physical activity.(2),(3),(4),(5) On the other hand, patients with a high internal locus of control, have lower pain frequency and intensity, decreased psychological issues, higher social integration, better compliance with treatment and medical advice, better health conditions, better self-management competency, and increased quality of life.(2),(3),(4),(5) Therefore, assessing the locus of control is essential as it influences a patient's attitudes, behaviors, and responses to interventions and treatments.(3),(4)

The management of MSK disorders promotes self-management strategies to improve clinical outcomes. A patient's disposition, such as their health locus of control, must be considered in the design of such rehabilitation programs to ensure patients have the resources to fulfill their goals. Clinicians caring for patients with a low internal health locus of control, should act as a coach to help these patients take control of their conditions. Increasing the internal locus of control has been documented to improve pain outcomes and health status.(4)

Assessment of the health locus of control in patients with MSK disorders can be done using the Multidimensional Health Locus of Control (MHLC), Form C, which demonstrates adequate reliability, test-retest stability, and validity in medical populations and in patients with different pain conditions (see Appendix J: Locus of Control).(1),(3),(6)

# References

1. Keedy NH, Keffala VJ, Altmaier EM, et al. Health locus of control and self-efficacy predict back pain rehabilitation outcomes. *Iowa Orthop J.* 2014;34:158-165.

2. Wahl AK, Opseth G, Nolte S, et al. Is regular use of physiotherapy treatment associated with health locus of control and self-management competency? A study of patients with musculoskeletal disorders undergoing physiotherapy in primary health care. *Musculoskelet Sci Pract.* 2018;36:43-47. doi:10.1016/j.msksp.2018.04.008

3. Bonafé FS, Campos LA, Marôco J, et al. Locus of control among individuals with different pain conditions. *Braz Oral Res.* 2018;32:e127. doi:10.1590/1807-3107bor-2018.vol32.0127

4. Musich S, Wang SS, Slindee L, et al. The association of pain locus of control with pain outcomes among older adults. *Geriatr Nurs.* 2020;41(5):521-529. doi:10.1016/j.gerinurse.2019.04.005

5. Wong HJ, Anitescu M. The role of health locus of control in evaluating depression and other comorbidities in patients with chronic pain conditions, a cross-sectional study. *Pain Pract.* 2017;17:52-61. doi:10.1111/papr.12410

6. Castarlenas E, Solé E, Racine M, et al. Locus of control and pain: validity of the Form C of the Multidimensional Health Locus of Control scales when used with adolescents. *J Health Psychol.* 2018;23(14):1853-1862. doi:10.1177/1359105316669860

# The Clinician

# Clinicians' Dispositions

—⊃⊂—

Attitudes and beliefs held by clinicians influence a patient's pain experience and management outcome. Clinicians influence a patient's understanding of the source and meaning of symptoms, as well as the expected prognosis. (1) There is strong evidence that a patient's beliefs are associated with their clinician's beliefs, and there is moderate evidence that patient and clinician fear-avoidance beliefs are also related.(1),(2) There is also strong evidence that clinicians commonly hold erroneous and unhelpful beliefs about MSK pain.(1),(3),(4),(5) Qualitative studies show that encounters with clinicians play an important role in the formation and perpetuation of unhelpful pain beliefs in patients.(1),(4),(6),(7),(8)

Unhelpful advice from clinicians to patients seeking care for MSK disorders, include activity avoidance to prevent further damage, avoidance of exercises to protect the damaged body part, and avoidance of dangerous postures and movements that contribute to body injury.(1),(5),(9),(10),(11),(12)

Clinicians can also convey erroneous information concerning the benefits and harms of treatments, screening, and tests. Clinicians rarely have accurate expectations of benefits or harms, with inaccuracies in both directions, but, more often, harms are underestimated, and benefits are overestimated.(13) Interventions might be oversold and overused if a clinician's expectations about intervention benefits are excessively optimistic or their knowledge of harms is insufficient.(13) Conversely, appropriate interventions may not be offered if clinicians underestimate the likely benefits or overestimate the harms.(13) Clinicians can believe that diagnostic imaging is an important tool to find the source of non-specific MSK disorders. They order diagnostic imaging to avoid missing a diagnosis that could lead to litigation, and to manage the patient's expectations.(14) Clinicians support the self-care of musculoskeletal disorders only as an adjunct to clinical management, and think it has only short-lived effects.(15)

Clinician beliefs can strongly impact the advice they give to their patients and can potentially reinforce unhelpful coping strategies.(1),(4),(5),(16) People who seek care when experiencing MSK disorders are more likely to have high levels of disability, high pain intensity, higher levels of fear, and more catastrophic beliefs.(8),(17),(18),(19) Given the impact of unhelpful beliefs and behavioral and emotional responses in MSK pain and disability (see chapters in section: The Patient), it is extremely important that physicians reflect on their own attitudes, beliefs, and experiences with pain. Clinicians have a significant and lasting impact on the attitudes, beliefs, and expectations of patients with MSK disorders. They need to take advantage of that opportunity to positively influence their patients, by understanding their patient's concerns, beliefs, and expectations, by reassuring patients about their disorder and prognosis, and by giving patients unambiguous messages about physical activity and work participation. Patients who feel valued and understood by their clinicians are more likely to achieve better recovery.

False beliefs and implicit bias can lead to racial and ethnic disparities in the assessment and treatment of pain.(20),(21) Many racial and ethnic minorities report provider-level bias and discrimination in relation to pain care.(20) Patients from minority groups have difficulty persuading clinicians about the impact of their pain, and feel that clinicians do not care about their pain experience.(20),(21). Higher rates of perceived discrimination lead to greater hopelessness and worse pain management outcomes.(20) Clinicians tend to rate patients from certain minority groups as having a higher pain tolerance, which leads to decreased prescriptions and dosages of pain medication. (20),(21),(22) People from minority groups undergo more scrutiny for potential drug abuse and are less likely to receive medication for their pain management.(20) Race continues to influence pain-related judgments. (20),(21),(22) These biases seem to be occurring at a subconscious level, rather than deliberately.(20),(21)

The ethnicity of the clinician can also influence a patient's assessment and treatment.(22) Pain ratings are comparable only between nurses and patients who share a cultural background.(22) A clinician's empathy towards their patient is higher between clinicians and patients of similar cultural backgrounds.(22) Clinicians need to become aware of subconscious biases they might have towards patients from minority populations, and apply strategies to overcome these false beliefs. Different strategies have been suggested to decrease racial bias: equal status contact, exposure to counter-stereotypic minority exemplars, competing on teams with a diverse racial or ethnic makeup, practicing the association of positive words with members of other racial or ethnic groups, and cultural competence training.(20),(22)

Appendix K provides clinicians with questions that can be used for self-reflection.

Appendix L addresses the discussion of imaging with patients who have non-specific low back pain.

# References

1. Darlow B, Dowell A, Baxter GD, et al. The enduring impact of what clinicians say to people with low back pain. *Ann Fam Med*. 2013;11(6):527-534. doi:10.1370/afm.1518

2. Darlow B, Fullen BM, Dean S, et al. The association between health care professional attitudes and beliefs and the attitudes and beliefs, clinical management, and outcomes of patients with low back pain: a systematic review. *Eur J Pain*. 2012;16:3-17. doi:10.1016/j.ejpain.2011.06.006

3. Bishop A, Foster NE, Thomas E, et al. How does the self-reported clinical management of patients with low back pain relate to the attitudes and beliefs of health care practitioners? A survey of UK general practitioners and physiotherapists. *Pain*. 2008;135(1-2):187-195. doi:10.1016/j.pain.2007.11.010

4. Caneiro JP, Bunzli S, O'Sullivan P. Beliefs about the body and pain: the critical role in musculoskeletal pain management. *Braz J Phys Ther*. 2021;25:17-29. doi:10.1016/j.bjpt.2020.06.003

5. Christe G, Nzamba J, Desarzens L, et al. Physiotherapists' attitudes and beliefs about low back pain influence their clinical decisions and advice. *Musculoskelet Sci Pract*. 2021;53:102382. doi:10.1016/j.msksp.2021.102382

6. Lin IB, O'Sullivan PB, Coffin JA, et al. Disabling chronic low back pain as an iatrogenic disorder: a qualitative study in Aboriginal Australians. *BMJ Open*. 2013;3(4):e002654. doi:10.1136/bmjopen-2013-002654

7. Bunzli S, Smith A, Schütze R, et al. Beliefs underlying pain-related fear and how they evolve: a qualitative investigation in people with chronic back pain and high pain-related fear. *BMJ Open*. 2015;5(10):e008847. doi:10.1136/bmjopen-2015-008847

8. Darlow B. Beliefs about back pain: the confluence of client, clinician and community. *Int J Osteopath Med*. 2016;20:53–61. doi:10.1016/j.ijosm.2016.01.005

9. Bunzli S, O'Brien P, Ayton D, et al. Misconceptions and the acceptance of evidence-based nonsurgical interventions for knee osteoarthritis. A qualitative study. *Clin Orthop Relat Res*. 2019;477(9):1975-1983. doi:10.1097/corr.0000000000000784.

10. Caneiro JP, O'Sullivan P, Smith A, et al. Implicit evaluations and physiological threat responses in people with persistent low back pain and fear of bending. *Scand J Pain*. 2017;17:355-366. doi:10.1016/j.sjpain.2017.09.012.

11. Caneiro JP, O'Sullivan P, Lipp OV, et al. Evaluation of implicit associations between back posture and safety of bending and lifting in people without pain. *Scand J Pain*. 2018;18(4):719-728. doi:10.1515/sjpain-2018-0056

12. Caneiro JP, O'Sullivan P, Smith A, et al. Physiotherapists implicitly evaluate bending and lifting with a round back as dangerous. *Musculoskelet Sci Pract*. 2019;39:107-114. doi:10.1016/j.msksp.2018.12.002.

13. Hoffmann TC, Del Mar C. Clinicians' expectations of the benefits and harms of treatments, screening, and tests: a systematic review. *JAMA Intern Med*. 2017;177(3):407-419. doi:10.1001/jamainternmed.2016.8254

14. Sharma S, Traeger AC, Reed B, et al. Clinician and patient beliefs about diagnostic imaging for low back pain: a systematic qualitative evidence synthesis. *BMJ Open*. 2020;10(8):e037820. doi:10.1136/bmjopen-2020-037820

15. Kovačević I, Kogler VM, Turković TM, et al. Self-care of chronic musculoskeletal pain - experiences and attitudes of patients and health care providers. *BMC Musculoskelet Disord*. 2018;19:76. doi:10.1186/s12891-018-1997-7

16. Colombo C, Salvioli S, Gianola S, et al. Traction therapy for cervical radicular syndrome is statistically significant but not clinically relevant for pain relief. A systematic literature review with meta-analysis and trial sequential analysis. *J Clin Med*. 2020;9(11):3389. doi:10.3390/jcm9113389

17. de Boer MJ, Struys MM, Versteegen GJ. Pain-related catastrophizing in pain patients and people with pain in the general population. *Eur J Pain*. 2012;16(7):1044-1052. doi:10.1002/j.1532-2149.2012.00136.x

18. Ferreira ML, Machado G, Latimer J, et al. Factors defining care-seeking in low back pain--a meta-analysis of population based surveys. *Eur J Pain*. 2010;14(7):747.e1-747.e7477. doi:10.1016/j.ejpain.2009.11.005

19. Mannion AF, Wieser S, Elfering A. Association between beliefs and care-seeking behavior for low back pain. *Spine (Phila Pa 1976)*. 2013;38(12):1016-1025. doi:10.1097/brs.0b013e31828473b5

20. Meints SM, Cortes A, Morais CA, et al. Racial and ethnic differences in the experience and treatment of noncancer pain. *Pain Manag*. 2019;9(3):317-334. doi:10.2217/pmt-2018-0030

21. Hoffman KM, Trawalter S, Axt JR, et al. Racial bias in pain assessment and treatment recommendations, and false beliefs about biological differences between blacks and whites. *Proc Natl Acad Sci U S A*. 2016;113(16):4296-4301. doi:10.1073/pnas.1516047113

22. Campbell CM, Edwards RR. Ethnic differences in pain and pain management. *Pain Manag*. 2012;2(3):219-230. doi:10.2217/pmt.12.7

# Communication

———∞———

Communication is the key to the patient-clinician relationship.(1) A patient-clinician relationship is more than signs and symptoms, and diagnosis and treatment. Patients might reveal fears, worries, or even secrets they have not disclosed to anyone before. Therefore, the clinical encounter must be a safe haven for patients that enables them to show their vulnerabilities and be authentic. For such a relationship, where patients feel that sense of security, open two-way communication is required. Effective communication will foster patient and clinician satisfaction by engendering trust, knowledge, regard, and loyalty.(2) These elements represent the foundation of the patient-clinician collaborative alliance.

Patient-clinician communication affects outcomes as well. The quality of communication during history-taking and management affects the frequency of visits, emotional health, and resolution of symptoms.(2) Communication about the effect of a treatment can affect the outcome. For example, negative pre-exercise information can lead to hyperalgesia after an exercise, whereas positive or neutral pre-exercise information yielded hypoalgesia.(3) In turn, high-quality communication involves the inclusion of the patient in the decision-making process, the provision of the patient with information programs, and the patient's own explanation and understanding of their disorder.(2)

Clinician communication is also positively correlated with patient adherence. A patient whose clinician communicates poorly has a 19% higher risk of non-adherence, compared to a patient whose clinician communicates well.(4) Clinicians need to be trained in communication skills to optimize adherence. A clinician with communication training has a 1.62 times higher chance of patient adherence.(4)

A favorable patient-clinician relationship is, therefore, paramount to maximize satisfaction, adherence, and outcomes. Interference in the patient-clinician relationship can arise from different factors that can put pressure on the relationship's foundations. Patient dispositions, clinician dispositions, patient-provider mismatch dispositions, and systemic dispositions can all contribute to an impaired patient-clinician relationship, and must be recognized and addressed in order to improve care (see Appendix M: Patient-Clinician Relationship).(2)

A key element of the clinical encounter is the interview. The interview is central to understanding patients and their problems. A disposition-based model of care requires a clinician to truly know each individual patient. This, of course, requires time to really listen to the patient and to meet the patient as a whole person. The clinical interview becomes a central component of the management. The patient biology, biography, history, and narrative are considered equally important information.(5) Listening to patient narratives is essential to understand their needs and values.(6) The patient's subjective description of their experience can provide key information for the causal story.(6) The discovery of a patient's concerns and addressing a patient's expectations leads to higher patient satisfaction.(7),(8) Effective communication, which produces a patient's context knowledge, needs, values, goals, and preferences about management, leads to a patient-centered partnership in management.(9) Patients are looking for a clinician who listens, genuinely cares, and sees them holistically and, therefore, can provide them with the best individual and personalized care.(10)

Medical education puts a lot of emphasis on biomedical information during the patient interview. Only a small part of a patient's disposition is recognized by such an interview technique. The biomedical information is of importance, of course, especially for identifying potentially life-threatening pathological processes, but is not enough to get a sense of the whole patient. The interview technique needs to integrate different aspects of a patient's life in order to get a meaningful picture. Clinicians need to use open-ended TED questions:

- **T**ell me your story.
- **E**xplain how you feel.
- **D**escribe what it's like.

Patients require time to answer these questions without interference from the clinician. The Common Sense Model (CSM) framework is a good tool to explore a patient's understanding of their disorders (see Appendix N: Common Sense Model).(11)

Effective communication considers the health literacy (capacity to obtain, process, and understand basic health information and services needed to make informed health decisions) of each individual patient. Limited health literacy negatively impacts clinician-patient communication.(12) Patients with limited health literacy use a more passive communication style, are less likely to engage in shared decision-making, and are more likely to report that interactions with their clinician are not helpful or empowering. (12) Therefore, clinicians need to adapt their communication style and the educational information provided by their patient's level of health literacy.

Clinicians with good communication skills will provide patients with effective elicitation (assessment of disease state and symptom burden, and uncovering of barriers to adherence) and explanation (conveying of test results and diagnoses, and discussion of treatment plan).(12) This, in turn, will lead to patient-clinician concordance, shared meaning and trust, respect, and therapeutic alliance.(12) Trust, respect, and therapeutic alliance leads to shared clinical decision-making and improved treatment adherence which, ultimately, yields better health outcomes (see Appendix O: Patient-Clinician Concordance).(12)

Verbal communication represents one of the most important social interactions between clinicians and their patients.(13) Slight differences in the wording of sentences might lead to different therapeutic outcomes.(13) Besides the power of verbal communication, nonverbal communication also plays a fundamental role in patient-clinician interaction. Sensory stimuli, such as vision and touch, represent the basis of nonverbal communication. (13) Facial expressions are an excellent source of information and play an essential role in communicating social intentions, from which people infer meaning.(13) Eye contact is another important aspect of social interaction and solicits attention and interest from the interacting persons.(13) Gestures and postures represent another key element of social interactions.(13) A person's behavior is affected by the perceived behavior of others (e.g. a person is more likely to rub their face if their interacting partner does so).(13) Intentions from someone can be inferred from observing one's gestures.(13) Nonverbal communication plays a fundamental role in the patient-clinician encounter. Therefore, clinicians need to be aware of the messages and intentions they transmit through facial expressions, eye contact, gestures, and postures.

# References

1. Honavar SG. Patient-physician relationship - Communication is the key. *Indian J Ophthalmol.* 2018;66(11):1527-1528. doi:10.4103/ijo._1760_18

2. Chipidza FE, Wallwork RS, Stern TA. Impact of the doctor-patient relationship. *Prim Care Companion CNS Disord.* 2015;17(5). doi:10.4088/pcc.15f01840

3. Vaegter HB, Thinggaard P, Madsen CH, et al. Power of words: influence of preexercise information on hypoalgesia after exercise-randomized controlled trial. *Med Sci Sports Exerc.* 2020;52(11):2373-2379. doi:10.1249/mss.0000000000002396

4. Zolnierek KB, Dimatteo MR. Physician communication and patient adherence to treatment: a meta-analysis. *Med Care.* 2009;47(8):826-834. doi:10.1097/mlr.0b013e31819a5acc

5. Anjum RL, Copeland S, Rocca E. *Rethinking Causality, Complexity and Evidence for the Unique Patient: A CauseHealth Resource for Healthcare Professionals and the Clinical Encounter.* New York, NY: Springer Publishing; 2020. https://www.springer.com/gp/book/9783030412388. Accessed Jan 15, 2021.

6. Rocca E, Anjum RL. Causal evidence and dispositions in medicine and public health. *Int J Environ Res Public Health.* 2020;17(6):1813. doi:10.3390/ijerph17061813

7. Berhane A, Enquselassie F. Patient expectations and their satisfaction in the context of public hospitals. *Patient Prefer Adherence.* 2016;10:1919-1928. doi:10.2147/ppa.S109982

8. Freilich J, Wiking E, Nilsson GH, et al. Patients' ideas, concerns, expectations and satisfaction in primary health care - a questionnaire study of patients and health care professionals' perspectives. *Scand J Prim Health Care.* 2019;37(4):468-475. doi:10.1080/0281 3432.2019.1684430

9. Lin I, Wiles L, Waller R, et al. Patient-centred care: the cornerstone for high-value musculoskeletal pain management. *Br J Sports Med.* 2020;54(21):1240-1242. doi:10.1136/bjsports-2019-101918

10. Kim K, Rendon I, Starkweather A. Patient and provider perspectives on patient-centered chronic pain management. *Pain Manag Nurs.* 2021;S1524-S9042(21)00036-9. doi:10.1016/j.pmn.2021.02.003

11. Caneiro JP, Bunzli S, O'Sullivan P. Beliefs about the body and pain: the critical role in musculoskeletal pain management. *Braz J Phys Ther.* 2021;25:17-29. doi:10.1016/j.bjpt.2020.06.003

12. Schillinger D. The intersections between social determinants of health, health literacy, and health disparities. *Stud Health Technol Inform.* 2020;269:22-41. doi:10.3233/shti200020

13. Benedetti F. Placebo and the new physiology of the doctor-patient relationship. *Physiol Rev.* 2013;93(3):1207-1246. doi:10.1152/physrev.00043.2012

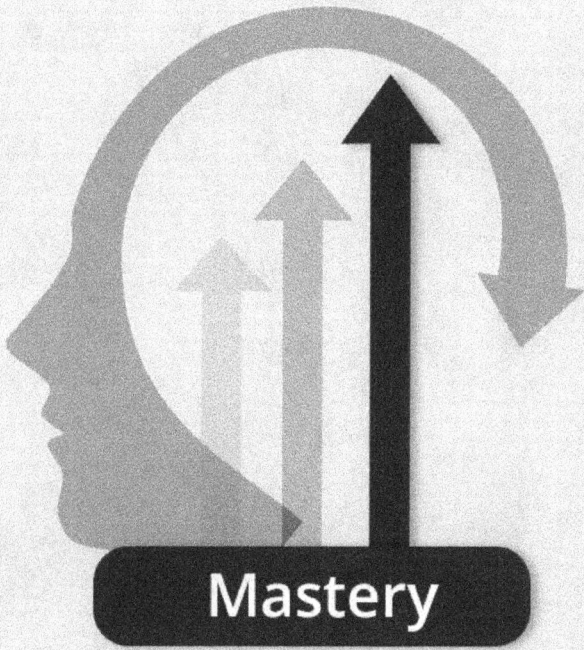
Mastery

Michael Vianin MSc DC

# Conclusion

# Bringing It All Together

Causality is a complex process that involves the manifestation of several dispositions in a particular person at a particular time. Manifestations result from the interaction of multiple dispositions and are, thus, complex. Dispositions can, together, produce an effect that cannot be produced by the single dispositions on their own; they are, in that sense, manifestation partners.(1),(2) No single disposition is the cause of the effect. Rather, all dispositions are causes since they all contribute to the effect.(1),(2).

This concept of manifestation partners, is well illustrated in this book as different causal powers will interact to produce an effect. For example, depression, poor sleep quality, poor metabolic health, and sedentarism will produce inflammation, which then impacts pain. Conversely, pain will impact depression, sleep quality, metabolic health, and the level of physical activity. Dispositions interact with each other to produce or modulate an effect. In turn, the effect alters the dispositions.

Contextual factors, the perception of self, psychological behavior (such as depression), reward mechanisms at play in pain catastrophizing, neuroimmune and neuroendocrine mechanisms active in metabolic health, and attitudes related to racial stereotypes, all share neuroanatomical pathways and neurophysiological processes. The different dispositions will, again, interact and impact each other, and will affect pain modulation. Conversely, pain will modify the dispositions.

A disposition-based model of care helps explain the difference in experiencing symptoms between patients. Patients with similar pathologies will experience different symptoms, depending on their disposition makeup.

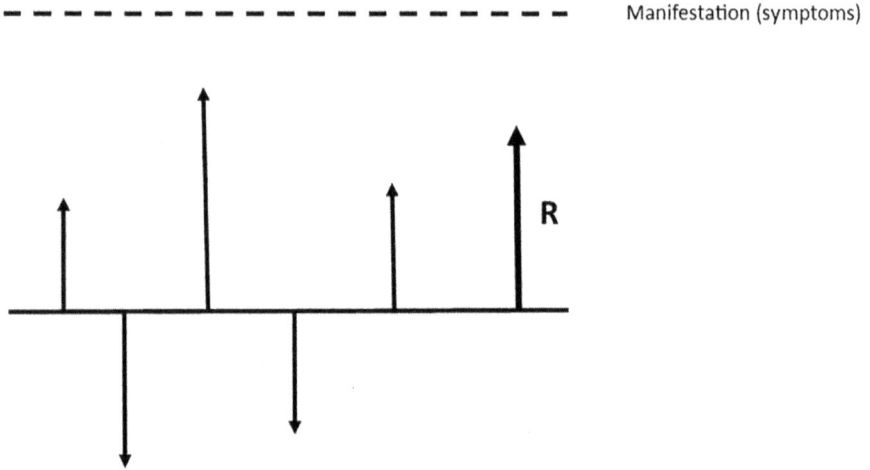

Manifestation (symptoms)

R

**Figure 21. Example A of the vector model.** Patient A experiences no symptoms.

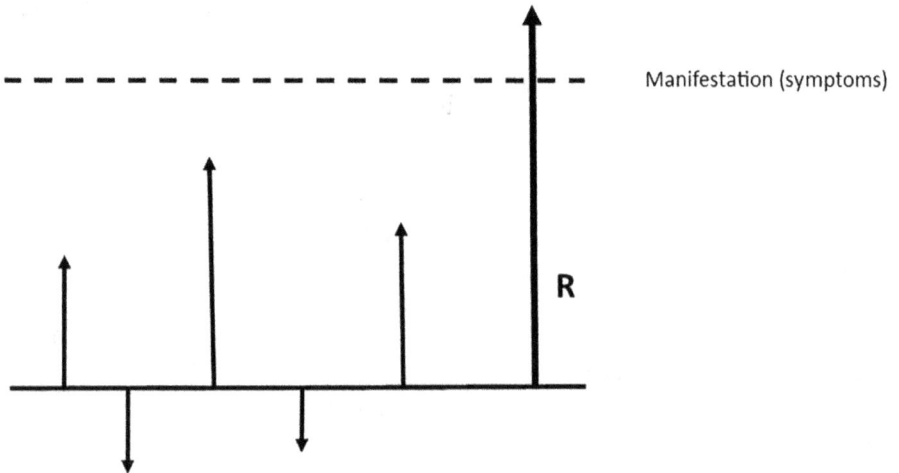

Manifestation (symptoms)

R

**Figure 22. Example B of the vector model.** Patient B experiences symptoms.

The same patients can experience their symptoms differently at any given time, depending on changes in their dispositions (e.g. less sleep, more stress, less physical activity). It is, therefore, critical to reassess a patient's dispositions, during flare-ups of their symptoms, or changes in their clinical presentation, to understand which changes in dispositions have occurred. Patients can become frustrated and anxious during pain flares. Understanding the nature of the flares will help clinicians explain why they happened and to reassure the patient. For example, pain-defined flares and self-reported flares have been shown to be increased by poor sleep quality in patients with LBP.(3)

The case of a 33-year-old woman with chronic right lateral elbow pain is presented here to illustrate how the modeling of the dispositionalism model can inform a patient's situation.

This patient had been suffering from right lateral elbow pain for years, with the pain becoming increasingly worse over time. She consulted her general practitioner, who diagnosed a lateral epicondylitis and prescribed her anti-inflammatory medication and some physiotherapy. The medication seemed to help a little for a while, but the effect did not last long. The physiotherapy did not help much. She was then referred to an orthopedic surgeon who injected her elbow with cortisone. This helped for about three weeks, after which the pain came back. The surgeon proposed operating on her elbow, which the patient refused.

The patient was eventually referred to another clinician by a friend. She expected to have a similar clinical experience to the one she previously had with the other clinicians she had visited for her elbow pain. She was surprised when the clinician asked her to tell her story about the pain and her life. She started by talking about the diagnosis and the different therapies and outcomes she had with them. The clinician then wanted to know how the pain affected her life and mood, and how she interpreted her pain. He wanted to know how emotions affected the pain and how the pain affected her emotionally. He took the time to know her as a person. For the first time, she felt someone genuinely listened to her and tried to understand her. The clinician showed her a couple of exercises to do at home and scheduled another appointment three weeks later.

The pain had gotten a little better by the second appointment, but was still quite disabling. The clinician then explained that a lot of factors play a role in the manifestation of pain and, if it was okay with her, he would like to ask her about some of these factors. Anything that made her uncomfortable would obviously not be addressed. They talked about her being an unemployed single mom of two, and all the stresses that situation involves. They also discussed her important weight gain over the last few years, due to stress overeating and the lack of any physical activity because she felt depressed, had to take care of her children by herself, and did not have the money to spend to go to a gym. The clinician explained to her how stress, obesity, depression, and financial difficulties impact her pain. He also motivated her to think about other factors that she felt could contribute to her pain.

During the third appointment, three weeks later, the patient felt that the therapeutic relationship was strong enough to share that she had been physically abused during her childhood and by her former boyfriend (the father of her children). She felt that the pain started when her former boyfriend began abusing her. The clinician explained to her how early childhood experiences and abuse later in life, both play an important role in chronic pain. He suggested she work with a psychologist to give her the tools to better deal with all that had occurred. The patient agreed and she started seeing a psychologist.

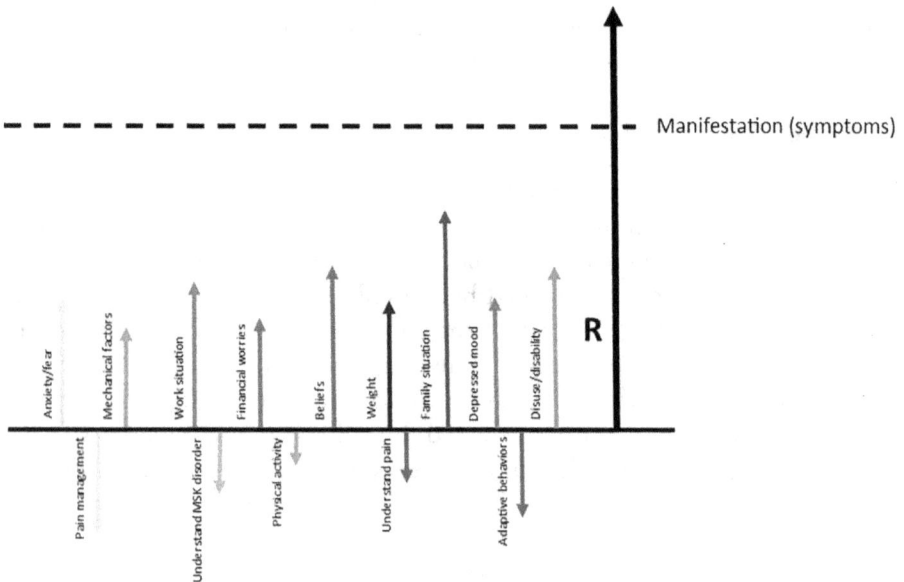

Figure 23. Patient's vector model third appointment.

The next appointment with the clinician was five weeks later. He noticed the patient looked more relaxed and happier. She was happier because the psychologist had helped her find some people to care for her children, and was working with her and a coach to find a job. She felt less pressure and stress and had started to go for walks with a friend once a week. The clinician was really impressed and explained how physical activity can help with pain and weight control. They talked about her weight gain and the clinician asked the patient if she would consider seeing a dietician. She agreed.

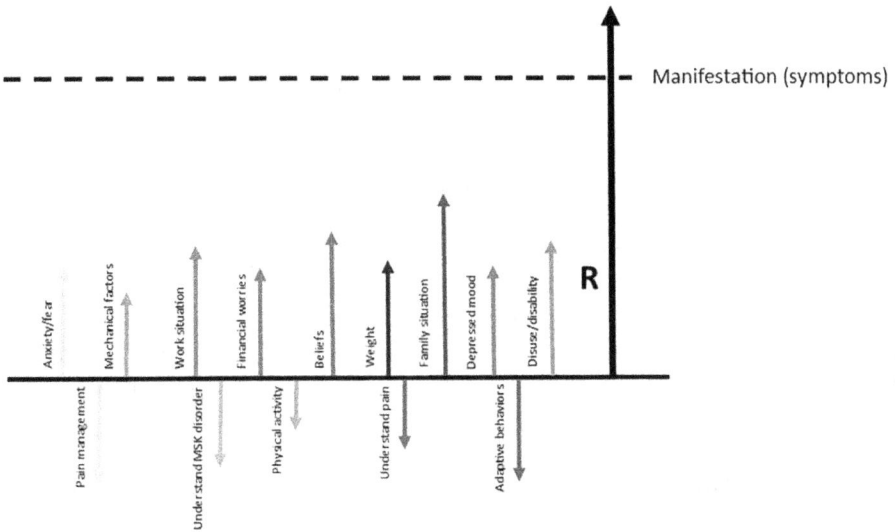

**Figure 24. Patient's vector model fourth appointment.**

By the next appointment, six weeks later, the patient was doing much better. Her pain was significantly improved, she had lost a couple of kilos, felt fitter, and she was going to start working in a couple of weeks. She was happy with all the changes made over the last few months and grateful for the guidance from the clinician.

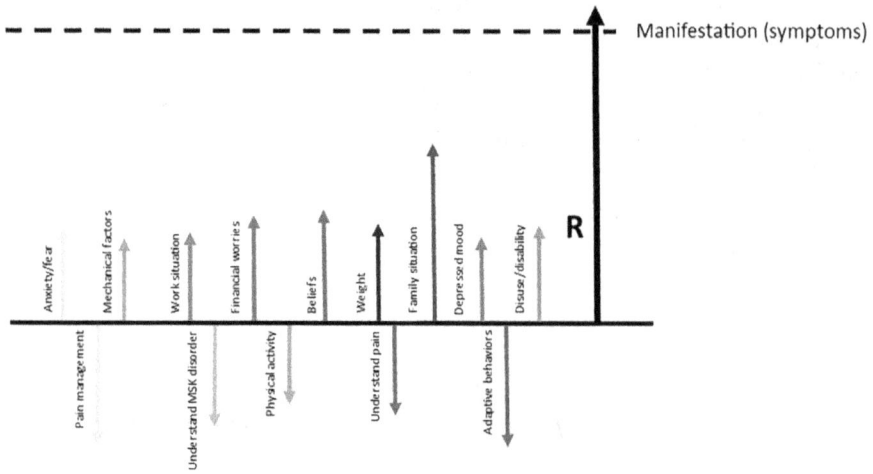

**Figure 25. Patient's vector model fifth appointment.**

Another six weeks later, the patient's pain was worse, even though she had lost more weight, was walking three times a week, was employed, and had help at home with her kids. The clinician asked the patient if she felt more fatigued, stressed, and depressed in the last couple of weeks. The patient said she had a difficult time over the last week, because she had to face her former boyfriend in a custody hearing for their children. She felt the pain got worse from that point. The clinician explained how the stress of facing her abusive former boyfriend impacted her pain, and reassured her that the flare-up was associated with that stress and anxiety. He recommended she contact her psychologist.

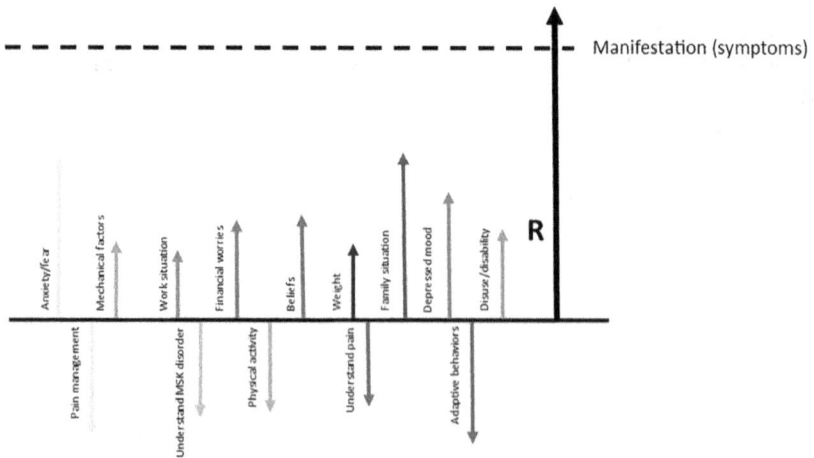

**Figure 26. Patient's vector model sixth appointment.**

Six weeks after the flare-up, the patient and the clinician met for the last time and the patient was doing well. The pain was almost totally gone and she felt well, having lost fifteen kilos, becoming physically active, working, and having settled her custody dispute.

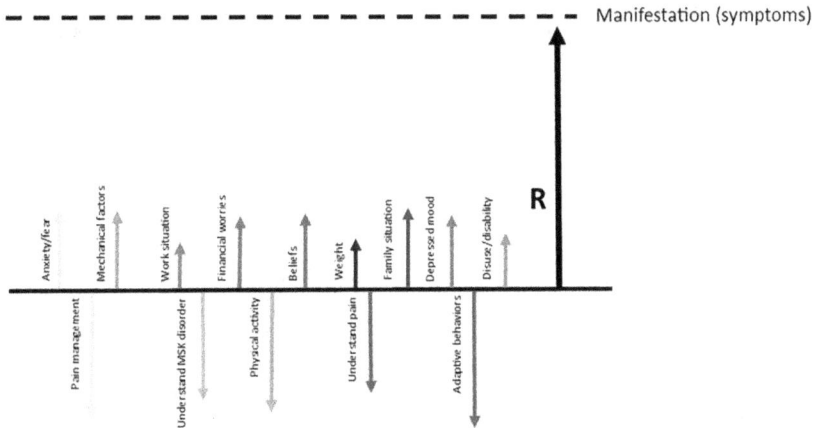

**Figure 27. Patient's vector model last appointment.**

A disposition-based model of care also provides a great tool for clinicians to understand which therapies might most benefit the patient. Therapies aimed at the more dominant dispositions are likely to provide the most benefit. The clinician then becomes a coach, who helps the patient understand the contributors to their clinical picture and which treatments are indicated. The patient, armed with that understanding, becomes a therapeutic partner who is actively involved in the decision-making of their care. A positive therapeutic alliance, which will positively influence management outcomes, is forged. Furthermore, the discovery of the dispositions influencing patients will give clinicians a tool to educate patients about the impact and the mechanisms of their dispositions on their health. This provides a unique educational opportunity to help patients better manage their condition.

The disposition-based model is applicable, not only to understand the intrinsic characteristics involved in the symptoms of the patient, but also for use in understanding the different parts of the clinical encounter. A vector model can be drawn to, for example, understand the factors at play for the therapeutic alliance. Dispositions, of both the clinician and the patient, that either promote or hinder a strong therapeutic alliance, can be visualized to see where mismatches are found and to find solutions to overcome them.

Understanding dispositions, their interactions, their effects, and the feedback loop from the effects to the dispositions, is essential to understand the patient experience and appropriately help patients take control of their symptoms. People going through pain, as described in The Common Sense Model chapter, try to gain control over the pain experience by making sense of it. Seeing the patient as a whole, and taking into consideration all the parts implicated in the pain experience, are the best ways to help a patient make sense of it and give them the most appropriate tools to gain control.

## References

1. Anjum RL, Copeland S, Rocca E. *Rethinking Causality, Complexity and Evidence for the Unique Patient: A CauseHealth Resource for Healthcare Professionals and the Clinical Encounter.* New York, NY: Springer Publishing; 2020. https://www.springer.com/gp/book/9783030412388. Accessed Jan 15, 2021.

2. Rocca E, Anjum RL. Causal evidence and dispositions in medicine and public health. *Int J Environ Res Public Health.* 2020;17(6):1813. doi:10.3390/ijerph17061813

3. Costa N, Smits E, Kasza J, et al. ISSLS PRIZE IN CLINICAL SCIENCE 2021: What are the risk factors for low back pain flares and does this depend on how flare is defined? *Eur Spine J.* 2021;30(5):1089-1097. doi:10.1007/s00586-021-06730-6

# Keep the Journey Going

The aim of this book was to look at the clinical encounter under a different set of lenses, and to motivate clinicians to think about the different dispositions, and their interactions during that exchange. For that purpose, it is essential that clinicians understand the mechanisms involved for the manifestation of causal powers.

This book is meant to be the starting point for discussions on dispositionalism in musculoskeletal care in classes, between colleagues, and with patients. A dedicated website, *www.mskcarethebook.com*, accompanying this book, will provide different resources to deepen understanding, and take the discussion concerning dispositionalism in musculoskeletal care further. All respectful and meaningful commentaries are welcome, as the journey to improve oneself is never-ending.

Michael can be contacted through the website to arrange interviews to further discuss the issues and concepts raised throughout this book. Presentations are also available and can be live, or in virtual, podcast, or radio formats. Journal interviews are also available on request.

Thank you for embarking on this journey of discovery.

# Appendices

————⊗————

## Appendix A: Clinical Encounter

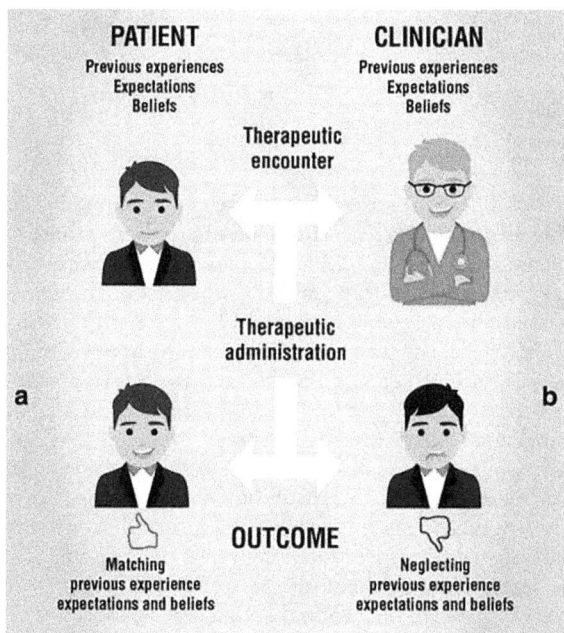

**Influencers of decision-making process.** The image presents: a the clinical situation in which meeting patient's expectation, previous experience and beliefs creates positive therapeutic outcomes; b the clinical situation in which ignoring patient's expectation, previous experience and beliefs creates negative therapeutic outcomes. Reprinted under the terms of the Creative Commons Attribution 4.0 International License from Rossettini G, Carlino E, Testa M. Clinical relevance of contextual factors as triggers of placebo and nocebo effects in musculoskeletal pain. BMC Musculoskelet Disord.

## Appendix B: Contextual Dispositions

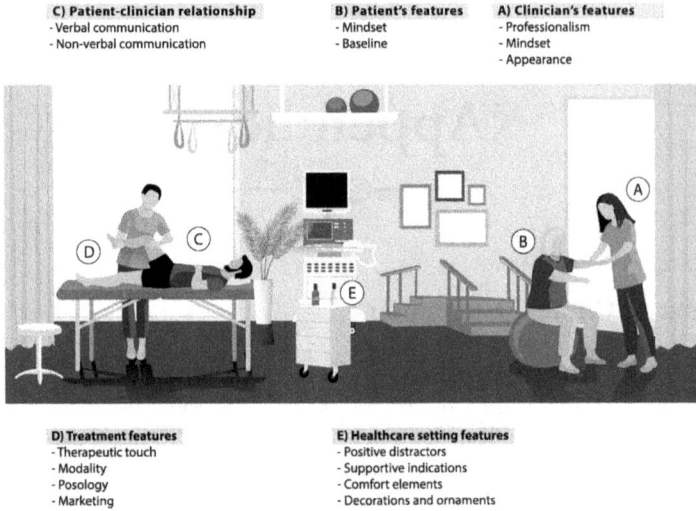

**C) Patient-clinician relationship**
- Verbal communication
- Non-verbal communication

**B) Patient's features**
- Mindset
- Baseline

**A) Clinician's features**
- Professionalism
- Mindset
- Appearance

**D) Treatment features**
- Therapeutic touch
- Modality
- Posology
- Marketing

**E) Healthcare setting features**
- Positive distractors
- Supportive indications
- Comfort elements
- Decorations and ornaments

**Contextual factors in clinical practice.** The following contextual factors were accepted as effective modifiers of treatment outcomes. **a** Clinician's features: professionalism (expertise, qualification, reputation, education, training); mindset (behavior, beliefs, expectation, previous experience); appearance (attire, uniform, white coat, trustworthiness). **b** Patient's features: mindset (expectation, previous experience, history of treatment, preference, desire, and emotion); baseline (level of symptoms, comorbidity, health condition, gender, age). **c** Patient-clinician relationship: verbal communication (positive message, tone of voice, active listening, suggestions of support and encouragement, language reciprocity, warmth, attention, care, empathetic interaction); non-verbal communication (eye contact, facial caring expression, smiling, posture, gestures, head nodding, forward leaning, open body orientation). **d** Treatment features: therapeutic touch (emotional, empathetic, affective); modality (level of invasiveness, open/overt application, observational/social learning); posology (personalized treatment, treatment delivered by the same clinician, cleanliness, adequate length of the consultation, punctuality, flexibility with patient's appointments, timely and efficient treatment, adequate frequency, duration and follow-up of therapy); marketing (brand, prize, novelty, rituality). **e** Healthcare setting features: positive distractors (natural lighting, low noise levels, relaxing and soft music, pleasing aromas, adequate temperature); supportive indications (highly visible and easy to read signs, parking information, accessible entrances, clear and consistent verbal or written directions, information desks and accessible electronic information); comfort element (windows and skylights, private therapeutic settings, good access to services, convenient clinic hours, location, parking, and available and approachable support staff); decorations and ornaments (nature artworks, green vegetation, flowers, water, plants, garden, color). Adapted under the terms of the Creative Commons Attribution 4.0 International License from Rossettini, G., Camerone, E.M., Carlino, E. et al. Context matters: the psychoneurobiological determinants of placebo, nocebo and context-related effects in physiotherapy. Arch Physiother.

# Appendix C: The Self

Table 1 | **Associations among psychosocial factors, physiology and health outcomes**

| Psychological and social factors | Physiological correlates | Health outcomes | Refs[a] |
|---|---|---|---|
| Anger, hostility | ↑ Adrenaline and noradrenaline<br>↑ Cardiovascular stress reactivity<br>↑ Systemic inflammation<br>↑ ACTH and CORT<br>↓ Parasympathetic cardiac control | ↑ Risk of CHD events in non-patients<br>↓ Prognosis in patients with CHD<br>↑ Risk of future stroke in non-patients | 215–223 |
| Depression | ↑ Adrenaline and noradrenaline<br>↑ Systemic inflammation<br>↑ ACTH and CORT<br>↓ Parasympathetic cardiac control | ↑ CHD mortality in patients with unipolar and bipolar depression<br>↓ Prognosis among patients with CHD<br>↑ Risk of CHD events in non-patients<br>↑ Cancer progression<br>↓ Survival in patients with cancer<br>↑ Risk of death in diabetes<br>↑ Risk of diabetes in non-patients | 80,216–219 |
| Anxiety | ↑ Systemic inflammation<br>↓ Parasympathetic cardiac control | ↑ CHD mortality in patients with anxiety disorders<br>↑ Risk of CHD events in non-patients | 213,220–223 |
| Chronic stress | ↑ ACTH and CORT in early phase<br>↓ ACTH and CORT in later phase<br>↓ Immune function<br>↑ Systemic inflammation<br>↑ Glucocorticoid resistance | ↑ Risk of CHD events and CHD-related death in non-patients<br>↓ Survival in patients with cancer | 224–226 |
| Positive emotionality | ↓ CORT<br>↓ Inflammatory responses to psychological stressors | ↓ Risk of death<br>↓ Risk of CHD-related death in non-patients<br>↓ Risk of death in patients with renal failure and HIV<br>↓ Risk of stroke<br>↓ Susceptibility to rhinovirus and influenza | 227–230 |
| Social support | ↓ Cardiovascular stress reactivity<br>↓ HPA axis stress reactivity<br>↓ Systemic inflammation | ↑ Survival after CHD event<br>↓ Risk of death<br>↓ Risk of CHD events<br>↑ Survival in patients with cancer<br>↓ Risk of cognitive decline | 231–233 |
| Social integration | ↓ Systemic inflammation | ↓ Risk of death<br>↓ Risk of future CHD events and CHD-related death in non-patients<br>↓ Risk of dementia and cognitive decline<br>↓ Risk of stroke<br>↓ Risk of developing respiratory infections<br>↑ Survival in patients with cancer | 234–239 |
| Acute stress reactivity | ↑ Adrenaline and noradrenaline<br>↑ HPA axis stress reactivity<br>↑ Cardiac contractility<br>↓ Parasympathetic cardiac control<br>↑ Blood pressure<br>↑ Heart rate<br>↑ Ventricular dysfunction<br>↑ Systemic inflammation | ↑ Risk of CHD events and CHD-related death in patients and non-patients<br>↑ Risk of hypertension | 58,240–243 |

ACTH, adrenocorticotropic hormone; CHD, coronary heart disease; CORT, cortisol; HIV, human immunodeficiency virus; HPA, hypothalamic–pituitary–adrenal.
[a]A general note on the advantages of prospective studies (such as those referenced here) is provided in Supplementary information S2.

**Associations among psychosocial factors, physiology and health outcomes**. ACTH, adrenocorticotropic hormone; CHD, coronary heart disease; CORT, cortisol; HIV, human immunodeficiency virus; HPA, hypothalamic–pituitary–adrenal. Reprinted with permission from publisher from Koban L, Gianaros PJ, Kober H, et al. The self in context: brain systems linking mental and physical health. Nat Rev Neurosci.

# Appendix D: Social History

## Table 4

Proposed topics for taking a more complete social history

---

**1. Individual characteristics**
• Self-defined race or ethnicity
• Place of birth or nationality
• Primary spoken language
• English literacy
• Life experiences (education, job history, military service, traumatic or life-shaping experiences)
• Gender identification and sexual practices
**2. Life circumstances**
• Marital status and children
• Family structure, obligations, and stresses
• Housing environment and safety
• Food security
• Legal and immigration issues
• Employment (number of jobs, work hours, stresses/concerns about work)
**3. Emotional health**
• Emotional state and history of mental illness (e.g., depression, anxiety, trauma, post-traumatic stress)
• Causes of recent and long-term stress
• Positive or negative social network: individual, family, community
• Religious affiliation and spiritual beliefs
**4. Perception of health care**
• Life goals & priorities; ranking health among other life priorities
• Personal sense of health or fears regarding health care
• Perceived or desired role for health care providers
• Perceptions of medication and medical technology
• Positive or negative health care experiences
• Alternative care practices
• Advance directives for cardiopulmonary resuscitation
**5. Health-related behaviors**
• Sense of healthy or unhealthy behaviors
• Facilitators of health promotion (e.g., behaviors among peers)
• Triggers for harmful behaviors and motivation to change (determined through motivational interviewing)
• Diet and exercise habits
• Facilitators or barriers to medication adherence
• Tobacco, alcohol, drug use habits
• Safety precautions: seatbelts, helmets, firearms, street violence
**6. Access to and utilization of health care**
• Health insurance status
• Medication access and affordability
• Health literacy and numeracy
• Barriers to making appointments (e.g., child care, work allowance, affordability of copayment, transportation)

---

**Proposed topics for taking a more complete social history.** Reprinted under the terms of the Creative Commons Attribution 4.0 International License from Andermann A. Screening for social determinants of health in clinical care: moving from the margins to the mainstream. Public Health Rev.

## Appendix E: Pain Catastrophizing

## <u>FACS</u>

Name:_____ ID #:_____ Date: ___/___/_____

**Instructions:** People respond to pain in different ways. We want to find out how you think and feel about your painful medical condition and how it has affected your activity level. Please think about how you have been over the past week, and circle one number between "0" and "5" from the scale below to answer each question.

**5 = Completely Agree**

**4 = Mostly Agree**

**3 = Slightly Agree**

**2 = Slightly Disagree**

**1 = Mostly Disagree**

**0 = Completely Disagree**

**Over the past week, how much do you agree with these statements about your painful medical condition?**

| | Completely Agree | Mostly Agree | Slightly Agree | Slightly Disagree | Mostly Disagree | Completely Disagree |
|---|---|---|---|---|---|---|
| 1) I try to avoid activities and movements that make my pain worse......................... | 5 | 4 | 3 | 2 | 1 | 0 |
| 2) I worry about my painful medical condition................... | 5 | 4 | 3 | 2 | 1 | 0 |
| 3) I believe that my pain will keep getting worse until I won't be able to function at all............................... | 5 | 4 | 3 | 2 | 1 | 0 |
| 4) I am overwhelmed by fear when I think about my painful medical condition............................. | 5 | 4 | 3 | 2 | 1 | 0 |
| 5) I don't attempt certain activities because I am fearful that I will injure (or re-injure) myself............................. | 5 | 4 | 3 | 2 | 1 | 0 |
| 6) When my pain is really bad, I also have other symptoms such as nausea, difficulty breathing, heart pounding, trembling, and /or dizziness...................................... | 5 | 4 | 3 | 2 | 1 | 0 |
| 7) It is unfair that I have to live with my painful medical condition....................................................... | 5 | 4 | 3 | 2 | 1 | 0 |
| 8) My painful medical condition puts me at risk for future injuries (or re-injuries) for the rest of my life................. | 5 | 4 | 3 | 2 | 1 | 0 |

Version 8, Rev. 1/30/2014

**Continue…..**

**Over the past week, how much do you agree with these statements about your painful medical condition?**

|  | Completely Agree | Mostly Agree | Slightly Agree | Slightly Disagree | Mostly Disagree | Completely Disagree |
|---|---|---|---|---|---|---|
| 9) Because of my painful medical condition, my life will never be the same………………………………… | 5 | 4 | 3 | 2 | 1 | 0 |
| 10) I have no control over my pain……………………… | 5 | 4 | 3 | 2 | 1 | 0 |
| 11) I don't attempt certain activities and movements because I am fearful that my pain will increase………………… | 5 | 4 | 3 | 2 | 1 | 0 |
| 12) It is someone else's fault that I have this painful medical condition…………………………………… | 5 | 4 | 3 | 2 | 1 | 0 |
| 13) The pain from my medical condition is a warning signal that something is dangerously wrong with me………… | 5 | 4 | 3 | 2 | 1 | 0 |
| 14) No one understands how severe my painful medical condition is………………………………………… | 5 | 4 | 3 | 2 | 1 | 0 |

**Start each of the following items with this statement: Over the past week, due to my painful medical condition I have avoided the following…**

|  | Completely Agree | Mostly Agree | Slightly Agree | Slightly Disagree | Mostly Disagree | Completely Disagree |
|---|---|---|---|---|---|---|
| 15) …strenuous activities (like doing heavy yard work or moving heavy furniture)………………………………… | 5 | 4 | 3 | 2 | 1 | 0 |
| 16) …moderate activities (like cooking dinner or cleaning the house)…………………………………………… | 5 | 4 | 3 | 2 | 1 | 0 |
| 17) …light activities (like going to the movies or going out to lunch)……………………………………………… | 5 | 4 | 3 | 2 | 1 | 0 |
| 18) …my full duties and chores at home and/or at work……… | 5 | 4 | 3 | 2 | 1 | 0 |
| 19) …recreation and/or exercise (things that I do for fun and good health)…………………………………………… | 5 | 4 | 3 | 2 | 1 | 0 |
| 20) …activities where I have to use my painful body part(s)… | 5 | 4 | 3 | 2 | 1 | 0 |

Total Score: _____

Version 8, Rev. 1/30/2014

**Fear-Avoidance Components Scale (FACS)**

**Appendix F: Depression**

## NICE guideline screening for depression

> During the last month, have you often been bothered by feeling down, depressed or hopeless?

> During the last month, have you often been bothered by having little interest or pleasure in doing things?

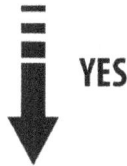

**YES**

> During the last month, have you often been bothered by feelings of worthlessness?

> During the last month, have you often been bothered by poor concentration?

> During the last month, have you often been bothered by thoughts of death?

**NICE Guidelines**

# Appendix G: Sleep Quality

## PITTSBURGH SLEEP QUALITY INDEX (PSQI)

**INSTRUCTIONS:** The following questions relate to your usual sleep habits during the past month only. Your answers should indicate the most accurate reply for the majority of days and nights in the past month. Please answer all questions.

1. During the past month, when have you usually gone to bed at night?
   USUAL BED TIME _____

2. During the past month, how long (in minutes) has it usually take you to fall asleep each night?
   NUMBER OF MINUTES _____

3. During the past month, when have you usually gotten up in the morning?
   USUAL GETTING UP TIME _____

4. During the past month, how many hours of actual sleep did you get at night? (This may be different than the number of hours you spend in bed.)
   HOURS OF SLEEP PER NIGHT _____

**INSTRUCTIONS:** For each of the remaining questions, check the one best response. Please answer all questions.

5. During the past month, how often have you had trouble sleeping because you...

|  | Not during the past month | Less than once a week | Once or twice a week | Three or more times a week |
|---|---|---|---|---|
| (a) ...cannot get to sleep within 30 minutes | ☐ | ☐ | ☐ | ☐ |
| (b) ...wake up in the middle of the night or early morning | ☐ | ☐ | ☐ | ☐ |
| (c) ...have to get up to use the bathroom | ☐ | ☐ | ☐ | ☐ |
| (d ...cannot breathe comfortably | ☐ | ☐ | ☐ | ☐ |
| (e) ...cough or snore loudly | ☐ | ☐ | ☐ | ☐ |
| (f) ...feel too cold | ☐ | ☐ | ☐ | ☐ |
| (g) ...feel too hot | ☐ | ☐ | ☐ | ☐ |
| (h) ...had bad dreams | ☐ | ☐ | ☐ | ☐ |
| (i) ...have pain | ☐ | ☐ | ☐ | ☐ |

(j) Other reason(s), please describe

_____

_____

| How often during the past month have you had trouble sleeping because of this? | ☐ | ☐ | ☐ | ☐ |

| | Very good | Fairly good | Fairly bad | very bad |
|---|---|---|---|---|
| 6. During the past month, how would you rate your sleep quality overall? | ☐ | ☐ | ☐ | ☐ |

| | Not during the past month | Less than once a week | Once or twice a week | Three or more times a week |
|---|---|---|---|---|
| 7. During the past month, how often have you taken medicine (prescribed or "over the counter") to help you sleep? | ☐ | ☐ | ☐ | ☐ |
| 8. During the past month, how often have you had trouble staying awake while driving, eating meals, or engaging in social activity? | ☐ | ☐ | ☐ | ☐ |

| | No problem at all | Only a very slight problem | Somewhat of a problem | A very big problem |
|---|---|---|---|---|
| 9. During the past month, how much of a problem has it been for you to keep up enough enthusiasm to get things done? | ☐ | ☐ | ☐ | ☐ |

| | No bed partner or roommate | Partner/ roommate in other room | Partner in same room, but not same bed | Partner in same bed |
|---|---|---|---|---|
| 10. During the past month, how much of a problem has it been for you to keep up enough enthusiasm to get things done? | ☐ | ☐ | ☐ | ☐ |

If you have a roommate or bed partner, ask him/her how often in the past month you have had...

| | Not during the past month | Less than once a week | Once or twice a week | Three or more times a week |
|---|---|---|---|---|
| (a) ...loud snoring | ☐ | ☐ | ☐ | ☐ |
| (b) ...long pauses between breaths while asleep | ☐ | ☐ | ☐ | ☐ |
| (c) ...legs twitching or jerking while you sleep | ☐ | ☐ | ☐ | ☐ |
| (d) ...episodes of disorientation or confusion during sleep | ☐ | ☐ | ☐ | ☐ |
| (e) Other restlessness while you sleep; please describe | ☐ | ☐ | ☐ | ☐ |

**Pittsburgh Sleep Quality Index (PSQI)**

## Appendix H: Physical Activity

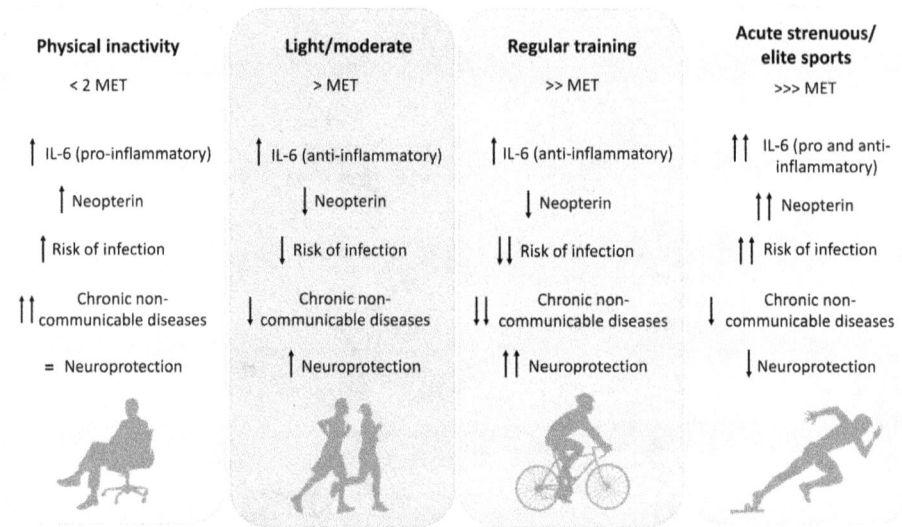

| Physical inactivity | Light/moderate | Regular training | Acute strenuous/ elite sports |
|---|---|---|---|
| < 2 MET | > MET | >> MET | >>> MET |
| ↑ IL-6 (pro-inflammatory) | ↑ IL-6 (anti-inflammatory) | ↑ IL-6 (anti-inflammatory) | ↑↑ IL-6 (pro and anti-inflammatory) |
| ↑ Neopterin | ↓ Neopterin | ↓ Neopterin | ↑↑ Neopterin |
| ↑ Risk of infection | ↓ Risk of infection | ↓↓ Risk of infection | ↑↑ Risk of infection |
| ↑↑ Chronic non-communicable diseases | ↓ Chronic non-communicable diseases | ↓↓ Chronic non-communicable diseases | ↓ Chronic non-communicable diseases |
| = Neuroprotection | ↑ Neuroprotection | ↑↑ Neuroprotection | ↓ Neuroprotection |

**Effects of physical inactivity and different intensities of physical exercise on the inflammatory response (IL-6 and neopterin) and health outcome (risk of infection, chronic non-communicable diseases and neuroprotection).** MET: metabolic equivalent of task. Reprinted with permission from author from Scheffer DD, Latini A. Exercise-induced immune system response: anti-inflammatory status on peripheral and central organs. Biochim Biophys Acta Mol Basis Dis.

# Appendix I: Self-Efficacy

Chronic Pain Self-Efficacy Scale (CPSS)

Name_____ Date_____

### Self-efficacy for pain management (PSE)

We would like to know how your pain affects you. For each question, circle the number that corresponds to how sure you are that you can do the tasks mentioned.

1. How confident are you that you can decrease your pain a little bit?

| 10 | 20 | 30 | 40 | 50 | 60 | 70 | 80 | 90 | 100 |
|----|----|----|----|----|----|----|----|----|-----|

Very confident        Moderately confident        Very confident

2. How confident are you that you can continue most of your daily activities?

| 10 | 20 | 30 | 40 | 50 | 60 | 70 | 80 | 90 | 100 |
|----|----|----|----|----|----|----|----|----|-----|

Very confident        Moderately confident        Very confident

3. How confident are you that you can keep your pain from interfering with your sleep?

| 10 | 20 | 30 | 40 | 50 | 60 | 70 | 80 | 90 | 100 |
|----|----|----|----|----|----|----|----|----|-----|

Very confident        Moderately confident        Very confident

4. How confident are you that you can make a small-to-moderate reduction in your pain by using methods other than taking extra medications?

| 10 | 20 | 30 | 40 | 50 | 60 | 70 | 80 | 90 | 100 |
|----|----|----|----|----|----|----|----|----|-----|

Very confident        Moderately confident        Very confident

5. How confident are you that you can make a large reduction in your pain by using methods other than taking extra medications?

| 10 | 20 | 30 | 40 | 50 | 60 | 70 | 80 | 90 | 100 |
|----|----|----|----|----|----|----|----|----|-----|

Very confident        Moderately confident        Very confident

**Self-Efficacy for physical function (FSE)**

We would like to know your self-confidence to perform some daily activities. For each question, circle the number that corresponds to how sure you are that you can do the tasks without help from others. Please consider what you can do on a daily basis, not isolated activities that require extraordinary effort.

1. How confident are you that you can walk 800 meters on flat ground?

| 10 | 20 | 30 | 40 | 50 | 60 | 70 | 80 | 90 | 100 |
|----|----|----|----|----|----|----|----|----|-----|

Very confident · · · · · Moderately confident · · · · · Very confident

2. How confident are you that you can lift a 5 kilos box?

| 10 | 20 | 30 | 40 | 50 | 60 | 70 | 80 | 90 | 100 |
|----|----|----|----|----|----|----|----|----|-----|

Very confident · · · · · Moderately confident · · · · · Very confident

3. How confident are you that you can perform a daily home exercise program?

| 10 | 20 | 30 | 40 | 50 | 60 | 70 | 80 | 90 | 100 |
|----|----|----|----|----|----|----|----|----|-----|

Very confident · · · · · Moderately confident · · · · · Very confident

4. How confident are you that you can perform your household chores?

| 10 | 20 | 30 | 40 | 50 | 60 | 70 | 80 | 90 | 100 |
|----|----|----|----|----|----|----|----|----|-----|

Very confident · · · · · Moderately confident · · · · · Very confident

5. How confident are you that you can shop for groceries or clothes?

| 10 | 20 | 30 | 40 | 50 | 60 | 70 | 80 | 90 | 100 |
|----|----|----|----|----|----|----|----|----|-----|

Very confident · · · · · Moderately confident · · · · · Very confident

6. How confident are you that you can engage in social activities?

| 10 | 20 | 30 | 40 | 50 | 60 | 70 | 80 | 90 | 100 |
|----|----|----|----|----|----|----|----|----|-----|

Very confident · · · · · Moderately confident · · · · · Very confident

7. How confident are you that you can engage in hobbies or recreational activities?

| 10 | 20 | 30 | 40 | 50 | 60 | 70 | 80 | 90 | 100 |
|----|----|----|----|----|----|----|----|----|-----|

Very confident · · · · · Moderately confident · · · · · Very confident

8. How confident are you that you can engage in family activities?

| 10 | 20 | 30 | 40 | 50 | 60 | 70 | 80 | 90 | 100 |
|----|----|----|----|----|----|----|----|----|-----|

Very confident · · · · · Moderately confident · · · · · Very confident

9. How confident are you that you can perform the work duties you had prior to the onset of chronic pain? (For homemakers, please consider your household activities as your work duties.)

| 10 | 20 | 30 | 40 | 50 | 60 | 70 | 80 | 90 | 100 |
|----|----|----|----|----|----|----|----|----|-----|

Very confident · · · · · Moderately confident · · · · · Very confident

### Self-efficacy for coping with symptoms (CSE)

We would like to know how you feel about your ability to control physical symptoms such as fatigue and pain. For each question, circle the number that corresponds to how sure you are that you can currently perform the activities or tasks mentioned.

1. How confident are you that you can control your fatigue?

| 10 | 20 | 30 | 40 | 50 | 60 | 70 | 80 | 90 | 100 |
|---|---|---|---|---|---|---|---|---|---|

Very confident — Moderately confident — Very confident

2. How confident are you that you can regulate your activity to be active without aggravating your physical symptoms (e.g., fatigue, pain)?

| 10 | 20 | 30 | 40 | 50 | 60 | 70 | 80 | 90 | 100 |
|---|---|---|---|---|---|---|---|---|---|

Very confident — Moderately confident — Very confident

3. How confident are you that you can do something to help yourself feel better if you are feeling blue?

| 10 | 20 | 30 | 40 | 50 | 60 | 70 | 80 | 90 | 100 |
|---|---|---|---|---|---|---|---|---|---|

Very confident — Moderately confident — Very confident

4. As compared to other people with chronic medical problems like yours, how confident are you that you can manage your pain during your daily activities?

| 10 | 20 | 30 | 40 | 50 | 60 | 70 | 80 | 90 | 100 |
|---|---|---|---|---|---|---|---|---|---|

Very confident — Moderately confident — Very confident

5. How confident are you that you can manage your physical symptoms so that you can do the things you enjoy doing?

| 10 | 20 | 30 | 40 | 50 | 60 | 70 | 80 | 90 | 100 |
|---|---|---|---|---|---|---|---|---|---|

Very uncertain — Moderately certain — Very certain

6. How confident are you that you can deal with the frustration of chronic medical problems?

| 10 | 20 | 30 | 40 | 50 | 60 | 70 | 80 | 90 | 100 |
|---|---|---|---|---|---|---|---|---|---|

Very confident — Moderately confident — Very confident

7. How confident are you that you can cope with mild to moderate pain?

| 10 | 20 | 30 | 40 | 50 | 60 | 70 | 80 | 90 | 100 |
|---|---|---|---|---|---|---|---|---|---|

Very confident — Moderately confident — Very confident

8. How confident are you that you can cope with severe pain?

| 10 | 20 | 30 | 40 | 50 | 60 | 70 | 80 | 90 | 100 |
|---|---|---|---|---|---|---|---|---|---|

Very confident — Moderately confident — Very confident

## Chronic Pain Self-Efficacy Scale (CPSS)

# Appendix J: Locus of Control

**Appendix 1** - Pain locus of control scale - C Form / Pain Locus Scale - C Form (PLOC-C)

Instructions for completing the scale (to be read to the patient, if applied as an interview): each item below is a belief statement about your pain that you may agree or disagree. Beside each statement is a scale that ranges from strongly disagree (1) to strongly agree (4). For each item we would like you to circle the number that represents the extent to which you agree or disagree with that statement. The more you disagree with a statement, the lower will be the number you circle. Please make sure that you answer EVERY

ITEM and that you circle ONLY ONE number per item. There are no right or wrong answers.

Scoring instructions for the scale (used by the examiner): The score on each subscale is the sum of the values circled for each item on the subscale (where 1 = strongly disagree and 4 = strongly agree). All of the subscales are independent of one another. There is no such thing as "total" score. The score is observed in each subscale so that the subscale with the highest score reflects the prevailing belief of the individual in the control of pain.

| Subscale | Possible range | Items |
|---|---|---|
| Internal locus of control | 6-24 | 1,6,8,12,13,17 |
| Chance locus of control | 6-24 | 2,4,9,11,15,16 |
| Doctors and health care professionals locus of control | 3-12 | 3,5,14 |
| Other people locus of control | 3-12 | 7,10,18 |

| | Strongly disagree | Slightly disagree | Slightly agree | Strongly agree |
|---|---|---|---|---|
| 1 If my pain worsen, it is my own behavior which determines how soon I will feel better again. | 1 | 2 | 3 | 4 |
| 2 As to my pain, what will be will be. | 1 | 2 | 3 | 4 |
| 3 If I see my doctor regularly, I am less likely to have problems my pain. | 1 | 2 | 3 | 4 |
| 4 Most things that affect my pain happen to me by chance. | 1 | 2 | 3 | 4 |
| 5 Whenever my pain worsens, I should consult a medically trained professional. | 1 | 2 | 3 | 4 |
| 6 I am directly responsible for my pain getting better or worse. | 1 | 2 | 3 | 4 |
| 7 Other people play a big role in whether my pain improves, stays the same, or gets worse. | 1 | 2 | 3 | 4 |
| 8 Whatever goes wrong with my pain in my own fault. | 1 | 2 | 3 | 4 |
| 9 Luck plays a big part in determining how my pain improves. | 1 | 2 | 3 | 4 |
| 10 In order for my pain to improve, it is up to other people to see that the right things happen. | 1 | 2 | 3 | 4 |
| 11 Whatever improvement occurs with my pain is largely a matter of good fortune. | 1 | 2 | 3 | 4 |
| 12 The main thing which affects my pain is what I myself do. | 1 | 2 | 3 | 4 |
| 13 I deserve the credit when my pain improves and the blame when it gets worse. | 1 | 2 | 3 | 4 |
| 14 Following doctor's orders to the letter is the best way to keep my pain from getting any worse. | 1 | 2 | 3 | 4 |
| 15 If my pain worsens, it's a matter of fate. | 1 | 2 | 3 | 4 |
| 16 If I am lucky, my pain will get better. | 1 | 2 | 3 | 4 |
| 17 If my pain takes a turn for the worse, it is because I have not been taking proper care of myself. | 1 | 2 | 3 | 4 |
| 18 The type of help I receive from the other people determines how soon my pain improves. | 1 | 2 | 3 | 4 |

**Pain locus of control scale - C Form / pain Locus Scale - C Form (PLOC - C)**

## Appendix K: Self-Reflection Questions for Clinicians

- What beliefs do I hold about the body and musculoskeletal pain?
- Where did these beliefs come from?
- What are my own experiences with pain?
- What was my coping response to the pain?
- What was my emotional response to the pain?
- Has this experience influenced the way I communicate with and manage my patients?
- Do I feel equipped to explore my patient's beliefs, and behavioral and emotional responses to pain?
- Am I aware of my own clinical biases?
- What stresses or frustrates me in clinical encounters?
- How do I respond to my patient's emotional distress or conflicting beliefs?

## Appendix L: Imaging Discussion Questions with Patients

- Did you explain the limited ability of lumbar imaging to locate the source of pain?
- Did you discuss the potential harms of imaging?
- Did you explore misperceptions expressed by your patient?
- Did you give your patient enough time to discuss their concerns and did they feel listened to, valued, and believed?

# Appendix M: Patient-Clinician Relationship

**Table 2. Patient Factors That Affect the Doctor-Patient Relationship and Suggested Solutions for an Impaired Relationship**

| Patient Factors | Strains on Relationship | Solutions |
|---|---|---|
| New patient | Trust: Not yet established<br>Knowledge: The doctor does not know the patient and vice versa<br>Loyalty: There has been limited opportunity to demonstrate loyalty | Regard: Maximize the patient's comfort and feeling of being liked<br>Knowledge: Take time to get to know the patient to maximize your knowledge of the patient |
| Poor prognosis | Trust: Medical knowledge and interventions may be exhausted<br>Regard: "Pathologic altruism," in which a physician may damage his or her relationship with a patient if the physician fails to recognize when treatment is futile, but continues to aggressively treat the patient, rather than focus on the patient's goals of care[19] | Trust: Ensure that the patient knows you have done everything possible<br>Loyalty: Do not abandon the patient<br>Regard: Find out what is important to the patient and work with him or her to maximize the quality of his or her final days[20,21] |
| Afflicted with a "frustrating" disease[a] | Trust: The doctor might not trust the patient<br>Regard: The patient and the physician might not like each other; the patient may feel judged; the doctor might have trouble being empathic | Loyalty: Make sure the patient knows that the physician is there for him or her<br>Trust: Educate oneself about the disease in question and the best ways to connect with the patient; create a dedicated team to support the treatment team for a challenging patient; in the case of substance abuse, studies have shown that patients in integrated care groups are more likely to remain abstinent compared to those in independent care groups[22]<br>Regard: Use motivational interviewing techniques to evaluate a patient's current willingness to change and to keep a patient's goals central to care |
| "Difficult" patient | Regard: The patient might dislike the physician; the doctor may dislike the patient | Knowledge: The physician should actively evaluate his or her feelings toward the patient ("autognosis" or self-knowledge), which allows the physician to use his or her own emotional reactions toward the patient as diagnostic information and allows the physician to thoughtfully change interactive styles with the patient to reduce tension[23] |
| Health literacy | Trust: The patient may not feel as though he or she has a basis on which to evaluate a doctor's competency<br>Knowledge: The doctor may provide educational materials that are above the patient's literacy level[24]<br>Regard: Misinformation may increase the risk of communication failures between the patient and the physician; using jargon may alienate a patient[25] | Knowledge: Physicians should evaluate their patient's health literacy and tailor the discussion to the patient's level[25]; the doctor should have the patient "teach back" the plan to ensure understanding |
| Family pressure[b] | Trust: A family may question a doctor's competence; the physician may not trust a family member to serve the patient's best interests<br>Knowledge: A family may know a patient better than the doctor does | Trust and knowledge: A doctor and other members of the care team (including nurses and social workers) should keep family members appropriately informed of a patient's status; frequent family meetings can be arranged<br>Regard: Demonstrate caring for the patient |

[a]Diseases that are generally considered difficult to treat (eg, substance abuse, substance-induced comorbidity, borderline personality disorder).
[b]Especially if the patient does not have decision-making capacity.

**Table 3. Provider Factors That Affect the Doctor-Patient Relationship and Suggested Solutions for an Impaired Relationship**

| Provider Factors | Strains on Relationship | Solutions |
|---|---|---|
| Physician burnout: state of detachment, emotional exhaustion, and lack of work-related fulfillment[26] | Trust: Lack of trust can lead to lower levels of patient satisfaction and to longer recovery times[27]; the behavioral consequences of burnout (eg, ineffective communication) also jeopardize trust and may damage the trust that patients have in a physician's competence<br>Knowledge: Attentive doctors are better able to understand both verbal and nonverbal communication[28]; therefore, burnout, which hinders attentiveness, prevents physicians from appreciating the needs of their patients, thus failing to identify their ailments<br>Regard: It is harder for emotionally exhausted physicians to show affection; when physicians are burned out, their patients are more likely to report that physicians use nonempathic statements[26]<br>Loyalty: Patients are less likely to return to a physician who fails to recognize their needs or who fails to regard them as individuals | Trust, knowledge, regard, and loyalty: All 4 elements are dependent upon physician well-being; strategies that improve a doctor's emotional wellness will optimize the doctor-patient relationship (eg, mindfulness meditation techniques, work-hour restrictions, participation in Balint groups, and programs to promote personal health [eg, exercise, nutrition, and sleep])[27-32] |
| Doctors in training or in early career | Trust: Patients may not trust a doctor's competence due to his or her young appearance or apparent lack of confidence<br>Loyalty: Patients might be reluctant to receive ongoing care from an inexperienced physician; patients may request care from an attending physician rather than from "a resident" | Trust: Take the time to explain your clinical reasoning to a patient to demonstrate competence<br>Knowledge: Get to know your patient<br>Regard: Demonstrate caring for your patient |
| Conflict on or with the treatment team | Trust: If a patient is given mixed messages by a team, faith in the team's ability to treat the condition may be lost<br>Knowledge: If team members fail to communicate effectively (eg, during poor "pass-offs"), then the doctor starting a shift may not know the patient sufficiently<br>Regard: Physicians may be distracted by team conflict and be unable to focus on the patient and his or her problem; doctors may displace frustration with the team onto the patient | Trust, knowledge, and regard: Use structured communication formats and regularly scheduled care-team meetings to improve teamwork[33]; include teamwork instruction as part of general medical education[34] |

Table 4. Patient/Provider Mismatches That Affect the Doctor-Patient Relationship and Suggested Solutions for an Impaired Relationship

| Patient/Provider Mismatches | Strains on Relationship | Solutions |
|---|---|---|
| Language barriers | Trust: Linguistic minorities report worse care than is provided to linguistic majorities[35]; physicians are less likely to share important medical information[36]<br>Knowledge: Doctors and patients may have more difficulty getting to know one another due to language barriers<br>Regard: Doctors are less likely to show empathy for a patient who is not proficient in the physician's language and are less likely to establish rapport[16,37] | Trust: Print educational handouts in the patient's language<br>Knowledge: Use skilled/trained interpreters rather than family members or members of the treatment team who speak "a little" of the patient's language<br>Regard: Encourage a greater expression of empathy |
| Cultural barriers | Trust: Patients may not trust Western medicine<br>Knowledge: Doctors may not understand the patient's health goals<br>Regard: Physicians may be judgmental about a patient who seeks complementary and alternative medical therapies | Knowledge: Whenever possible, use interpreters who act as cultural ambassadors as well as language interpreters; use frameworks, such as Kleinman's 8 questions,[10] to elicit the patient's explanatory model; encourage physician participation in global health initiatives[38]<br>Regard: Acknowledge and incorporate traditional practices whenever possible[39-41] |
| Locus of control[a] | Knowledge: Patients may know themselves better than the doctor knows them and therefore know the best treatment<br>Regard: Power struggles may damage rapport | Knowledge and regard: A mutual participation model can be employed[3] |

[a]Locus of control (ie, Who is ultimately making the decisions?).

Table 5. Systemic Factors That Affect the Doctor-Patient Relationship and Suggested Solutions for an Impaired Relationship

| Systemic Factors | Strains on Relationship | Solutions |
|---|---|---|
| Time constraints | Trust: Doctors may not have or make the time to explain their reasoning to engender the patient's trust<br>Knowledge: There is less time for the physician and the patient to get to know one another<br>Regard: There is less time to establish rapport<br>Loyalty: Patients are less likely to be loyal to a doctor if they have not developed positive regard | Trust, knowledge, regard, and loyalty: Develop strategies to increase workplace efficiency, leaving time for physicians to explain their reasoning, to know patients, and to establish rapport; by using prescreening forms and questionnaires while the patient is in the waiting room or by using simple technologies (eg, walkie-talkies to communicate with medical assistants and other support staff), more time can be devoted to patient care[42] |
| Space/room | Knowledge: If the space is not private, physicians may be reluctant to ask certain questions, which limit their ability to know the patient; additionally, patients may be reluctant to confide in doctors if they do not feel the conversation is private<br>Regard: Busy and uncomfortable clinics may make it harder for the doctor and patient to connect | Knowledge: Whenever possible, take the patient into a private room to ask questions |
| High patient-provider ratio[a] | Knowledge: Patients may feel like they are objects being discussed, rather than as equals participating in their own care; they may not feel as though they know all of the team members and what their roles are<br>Regard: There may be too many people with whom to establish rapport | Trust: Explain each team member's role and how they contribute to the patient's care<br>Knowledge and regard: Whenever possible, limit the number of physicians who round on a patient at one time; in teaching hospitals, where this is not always possible, team members should introduce themselves to the patient outside of rounds to establish rapport and to know the patient |
| Urgent care setting (eg, emergency department, clinic) | Knowledge: The doctor and the patient may not know each other<br>Regard: The patient and the physician may be less inclined to invest effort in establishing rapport if they know they will not see each other again<br>Loyalty: Clinics may not be set up for longitudinal care (eg, in the emergency department) | Knowledge: The doctor can learn about a patient's history by calling the patient's prior providers and informing the patient that the providers will receive the results of any testing<br>Regard: Take the time to establish rapport and to make the patient feel comfortable whenever possible<br>Loyalty: Set up follow-up appointments with established providers before discharging the patient |
| Cost | Regard: The patient may harbor resentment about medical bills<br>Loyalty: The patient may be reluctant to see a doctor due to financial concerns | Knowledge: Make the cost of care a part of the routine conversation with the patient; for example, one can discuss a patient's financial concerns, connect a patient to a social worker or to other financial resources, work with a patient on treatment plans he or she feels are affordable, and prescribe generics when available |
| Documentation burden | Knowledge: Physicians may spend much of the visit making sure all the necessary computer boxes are checked rather than getting to know the patient as a person; having a computer between the patient and the doctor also makes it hard for the patient to feel like he or she knows the doctor<br>Regard: Physicians may spend much of the visit facing the computer screen rather than the patient, which may make the patient feel as though the doctor does not care about him or her as a person; the amount of paperwork and documentation that is often required also enhances physician burnout, making it harder for the physician to demonstrate empathy and caring | Several time-saving strategies can be employed to reduce the amount of time spent on documentation and increase the time available for physicians to spend with patients<br>Embrace technology: personal mobile computers can improve provider efficiency[43]<br>Use dictation software to speed note-writing<br>When appropriate, write a note collaboratively with the patient during the visit; if using this approach, either turn the screen so that the patient can see it as well or arrange seats so that the physician can maintain eye contact with the patient while he or she is typing the notes |

[a]Refers specifically to teaching rounds, wherein a large team of providers visits a patient as a group.

**Factors that influence the clinician-patient relationship.** Reprinted with permission from publisher from Chipidza FE, Wallwork RS, Stern TA. Impact of the doctor-patient relationship. Prim Care Companion CNS Disord.

## Appendix N: Common Sense Model (CSM)

| CSM constructs | | Example questions |
|---|---|---|
| | Interpretation | Tell me your story.Put me in your shoes and tell me how your pain feels? How has the pain impacted on you?How has the pain impacted your home/work/social life? |
| Representation | Identity | What is your understanding of your problem?What do you think is going on in your body?Have you received a diagnosis for your pain? How do you see it?Have you had scans for this condition? What is your understanding of the scan results?When you have pain what do you think it means? |
| | Cause | What is your understanding of the cause/s of your pain? |
| | Consequences | How does the pain impact on your life (physical, work, social etc.)? What do you think will happen if you perform a movement or activity that you avoid? |
| | Control/Curability | How much control do you feel you have over your pain?If so, how do you control your pain?How confident are you to do the things that you value? Can you prevent your pain from flaring up?Can you control your pain once it has flared up? |
| | Timeline | How long do you expect your pain will last?Can you see yourself getting back to work, sport or other valued activities?How hopeful are you for the future? How do you see your future? Where do you see yourself in 3 months/1 year?Do you think your pain will get better? |
| Behavioral response | Action | When you have pain, what do you do?What do you do when faced with a threatening movement or activity?Do you avoid important activities because of your pain?Do you modify how you do important activities because of your pain?Why do you think you shouldn't bend/lift/run/social/work activities etc.?Would your life look different if you didn't have pain?What do you think it will take to get better? |
| | Appraisal | Is this action effective? Has it worked for you?Tell me about your goalsWhat do you think you need to achieve your goals?Is this action aligned with your goals? |
| Emotional response | Emotion | How does the pain make you feel?How do you feel about losing the ability to do things you love?Does this pain get you down?Do you worry about your pain?Do you fear your pain or doing damage to yourself?How do others you care about see you? |
| | Coherency | How much does your pain make sense to you? |

**How to explore patients' understanding of pain using the CSM framework.** Reprinted with permission from publisher from Caneiro JP, Bunzli S, O'Sullivan P. Beliefs about the body and pain: the critical role in musculoskeletal pain management. Braz J Phys Ther.

# Appendix O: Patient-Clinician Concordance

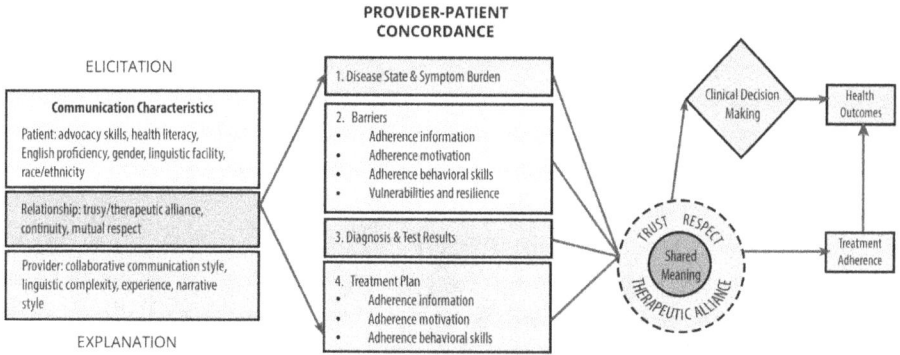

**Model for successful communication with patients in the clinical encounter.** Reprinted with permission from publisher from Schillinger D. The intersections between social determinants of health, health literacy, and health disparities. Stud Health Technol Inform.

www.ingramcontent.com/pod-product-compliance
Lightning Source LLC
Chambersburg PA
CBHW070921270326
41927CB00011B/2666